about the author

Judy Chapman was born in 1967 and grew up commuting
between Melbourne and Byron Bay. She has always had a
passion for natural healing and in 1990 she co-founded and created
Sanctum Pure Body Products — a range of natural, petrochemical-
free hair and skin products. Based on the principles of
aromatherapy, the range was produced in Byron Bay. She has also
studied a variety of alternative therapies and healing, including
macrobiotics at the Kushi Institute of Amsterdam.

Judy Chapman is now working on a variety of aromatherapy-
related projects and is also Public Relations/Communications
Manager for Planet Ark, Australia's largest environmental education
organisation. This is her first book.

photography by Robert Reichenfeld

styling by Anna-Marie Bruechert

Aromatherapy

recipes for your oil burner

judy chapman

HarperCollins*Publishers*

HarperCollins*Publishers*

First published in Australia in 1998
by HarperCollins*Publishers* Pty Limited
ACN 009 913 517
A member of HarperCollins*Publishers* (Australia) Pty Limited Group
http://www.harpercollins.com.au

HarperCollins*Publishers*
25 Ryde Road, Pymble, Sydney, NSW 2073, Australia
31 View Road, Glenfield, Auckland 10, New Zealand
77–85 Fulham Palace Road, London W6 8JB, United Kingdom
Hazelton Lanes, 55 Avenue Road, Suite 2900, Toronto, Ontario M5R 3L2
and 1995 Markham Road, Scarborough, Ontario M1B 5M8, Canada
10 East 53rd Street, New York NY 10032, USA

National Library Cataloguing-in-Publication data:

Chapman, Judy, 1967–.
 Aromatherapy recipes for your oil burner.
 Includes index.
 ISBN 0 7322 5914 2.
 1. Aromatherapy – Popular works. 2. Aromatherapy.
 I. Title.
668.542

Haikus on pages xvi, 23, 34, 76, 89, 111, 133, 141 and 149 are reproduced from *A Haiku Garden* by Stephen
Addiss with Fumiko and Akira Yamamoto with kind permission of the publishers, Weatherill, Inc., New York.
The haiku on page 123 is reproduced from *A Long and Rainy Season*, 1994, edited by Leza Lowitz, Miyuki
Aoyama and Akemi Tomioka with kind permission of the publishers, Stone Bridge Press, Berkeley, CA.

Cover and internal photography by Robert Reichenfeld
Styling by Anna-Marie Bruechert
Set in Futura 11/18
Printed in Singapore by Kyodo Printing Co. on 115gsm Matt Art

5 4 3 2 1
02 01 00 99 98

contents

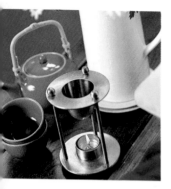

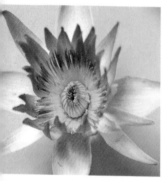

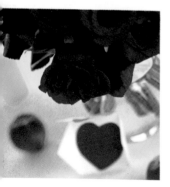

about aromatherapy

Aromatherapy is the use of pure essential oils, and is an absolutely beautiful way to celebrate life and help heal yourself, your family and your environment. The art of aromatherapy is used in many ways: in vaporisation, massage, inhalations, compresses, cosmetics and even pharmaceutical medicines. Sourced from nature, pure essential oils have the power to bring calm and joy and to rejuvenate and nourish our mind, body and spirit.

Human beings are extremely vulnerable to scent, and we will often react to a smell emotionally before becoming aware of it physically. As with our other senses, smells can affect our moods in both positive and negative ways, and may invoke both pleasant and painful memories. A lovely fragrance will lift our spirits, whereas an objectionable odour can bring us down. In scientific terms, this is because smell sends a direct message to the limbic system, the part of the brain that governs emotions.

Essential oils are sometimes called the 'life force' of plants. The oils are extracted from various parts of the plant: the roots, leaves, flowers, bark and fruit; and have been used for centuries to heal both animals and human beings. They were also used for spiritual as well as physical purposes: priests would burn myrrh and juniper to enhance the spiritual awareness of their congregations, and in ancient Egypt, Cleopatra was known to use rose oil as an aphrodisiac. Even up until a hundred years ago, humans primarily used plants, herbs and essential oils to heal themselves. It is only recently that humans have begun to manufacture synthetic drugs which, despite their medicinal benefits, also carry the danger of both known and as yet undiscovered side effects.

Essential oils are usually extracted from plants by steam distillation. The oil-giving part of the plant is placed inside a stainless steel distillation vat and the extreme pressure of the steam around the vat breaks down the plant material, releasing the essential oil from the plant cells. When cooled, the

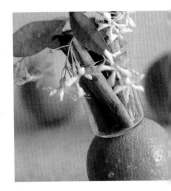

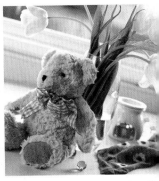

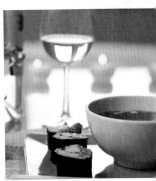

oils separate naturally from the water. The residual water is used for cosmetic purposes and is known as 'floral water' (orange blossom water or rosewater are two well-known types of floral water). Floral water makes a delicious hydrating and refreshing splash for the face and body. For the most part, essential oils, if packaged properly in dark glass and stored in a cool, dry area, will retain their aroma for years. The quality of an essential oil depends primarily on the growing conditions of the plant: soil, weather and the timing of the harvest will all influence the fragrance, colour and potency of the extracted essential oil.

Aromatherapy is just one way we can learn to heal ourselves. The key to living a fulfilled life is to nourish and balance ourselves on all levels, including eating a balanced diet with organic fruit and vegetables and drinking pure water, and choosing forms of exercise that best suit your body and lifestyle. And it's just as important to be spiritual, creative and to have fun. We choose and create our own lives — learning our lessons, becoming stronger through these experiences, resolving past conflicts and realising our highest potential. We are all wonderful beings, and we each carry special gifts and varied experiences to share with each other.

The recipes in this book have been created purely for vaporising. Vaporisation occurs when a few drops of an essential oil are added to warm water, heated in an oil burner, or vaporiser. The heat causes the oils to evaporate, filling the atmosphere with their exquisite healing aromas. These wonderful fragrances generate a natural feeling of wellbeing and influence the range of emotional and physical conditions that touch us as we go about our daily lives.

beginning aromatherapy

There are several things you will need in your aromatherapy starter kit:

- a vaporiser or oil burner
- small tea-light candles
- essential oils of your choice
- a box and a cool, dry place for storing your oils

A vaporiser, or oil burner, is a two-tiered structure with a dish at the top to hold water and the essential oils, and a surface below to hold a tea-light candle. It is preferable to choose a vaporiser with a ceramic dish so that the oils do not permeate the dish, permanently impregnating it with their aroma. Fill the ceramic dish with water and heat it by placing a lighted candle underneath it. The best tea-light

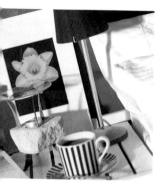

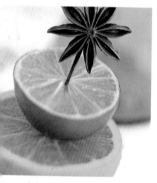

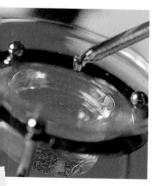

candles are made of beeswax and last for up to eight hours. Once the water is warm, add the required number of drops of essential oil to its surface.

Always buy aromatherapy oils that are marked as being 100 per cent pure. There are many perfume oils around that are not essential oils and do not have the healing properties of pure essential oils. For example, if the label on a bottle of Ylang Ylang oil reads: 'Ylang Ylang aromatic or perfume oil', this is not an essential oil. However, if the label reads: '100% pure Ylang Ylang essential oil', this would be the correct choice. Some oils, however, like Rose, Jasmine and Chamomile, are extremely expensive and are usually sold diluted at five per cent in a carrier oil. As long as it is clear that the essential oil is pure, its aromatherapeutic use will be effective.

Essential oils are easily affected by light, so always buy oils that have been packaged in dark glass. Do not under any circumstances store essential oils in plastic; the oils will cause the plastic to deteriorate and the oils themselves will lose their therapeutic properties. Similarly, keep your oils away from heat and moisture (for example, do not store them in your bathroom). The best place to store your oils is in a wooden box in a cool, dry place. A wooden box also makes the ideal travelling container.

The recipes in this book are intended as a guide only. One of the greatest pleasures of aromatherapy is creating your own personal blends. Experimenting with oils that you like, and studying their properties, will give you the confidence to create your own uplifting atmosphere at work and at home.

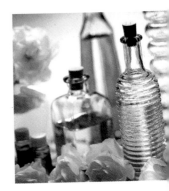
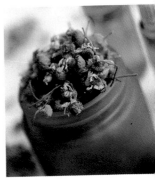
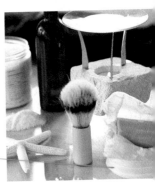

some important points to remember when using essential oils

There are certain precautions that must be followed when using essential oils. Some essential oils are harmful to pregnant women, so make sure that before using each oil you check its properties in the glossary at the back of this book.

Here are some key points to remember when using essential oils:

- Keep oils out of the reach of children.
- Never apply directly on to the skin.
- Never take internally.
- Never apply essential oils when sunbathing.
- Keep essential oils away from the eyes. (If you do accidentally get oil in your eyes, splash immediately with tepid water or milk. Seek medical advice if discomfort persists.)
- Discontinue the use of essential oils immediately if you suffer an allergic reaction, and seek professional advice.
- Never dilute more than a total of eight drops of essential oils in water for vaporisation, unless advised otherwise by a qualified aromatherapist.
- Always purchase essential oils that are 100 per cent pure.
- Always purchase essential oils that are packaged in dark glass and stored away from intense heat or light.

acknowledgements

This book is the completion of a dream I have held in my heart since I was very young. There are many people I need to thank: Kayti Denham for her help with the research and creation of these beautiful recipes. My precious family who have kept my spirit alive and joyous — my sister Jessie, you are my soul sister, my constant inspiration; my mother CC for your incredible support, love and freedom; and my father Daryl — our meeting again has made me complete. Kevin Purtill for all your love — I value your friendship more than ever! Jack Allanach for your editing contribution and for Sourabh — together you bring out the laughter in me! Helen Littleton, Nicola O'Shea and Judi Rowe from HarperCollins for all your creativity and direction. All the people who have come in and out of my life with warmth and understanding — Khim Newland, Maya Sweeney, Arthur Lawrence, David Rock, Jaya, Varij, the Tuer family, Margaret Stoops, Grandma and Grandpa. And thanks to Sanctum, Planet Ark, the Sydney School of Zi Ran Qigong and the Kushi Institute for valued learning experiences and knowledge.

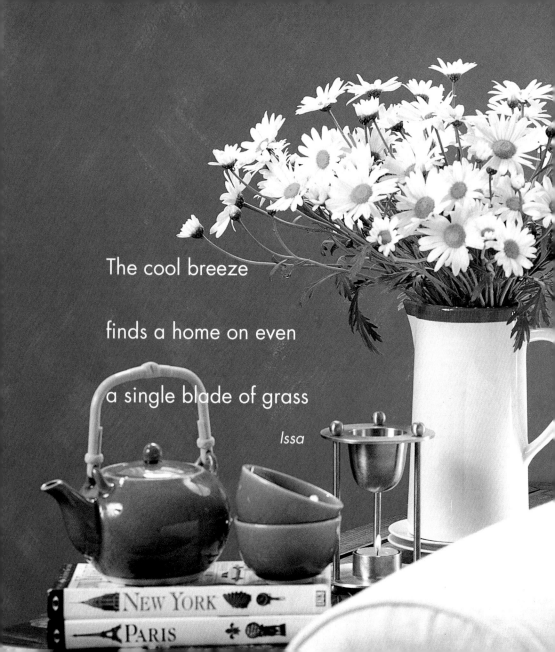

The cool breeze

finds a home on even

a single blade of grass

Issa

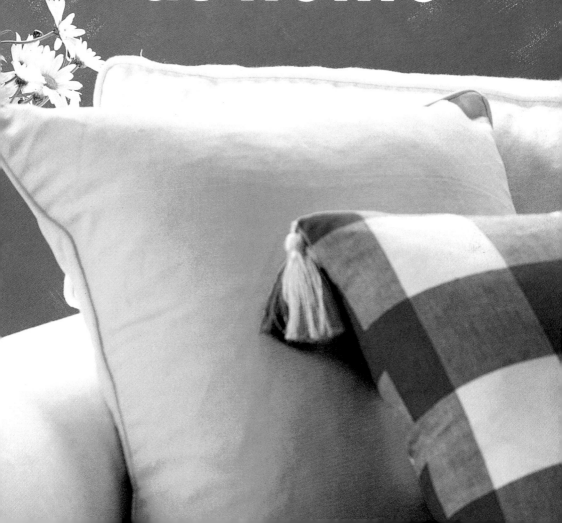

at home

Whether you live in a tent, flat or mansion, home is a haven where you can be completely open and express yourself comfortably. Your home is said to reflect your state of being. It can be a place of warmth, love and peacefulness, where you can enjoy lively and joyful interaction with family and friends or a place where you can retreat and enjoy being alone. The recipes in this section have been created to help create an atmosphere of comfort and happiness in your home.

moving in

Moving into a new home can be joyfully exhausting, but it's also the perfect opportunity to create a new secure and cosy sanctuary where you can replenish yourself when the world gets too crazy. This blend combines mystical and soothing qualities to fill your new home with an air of quiet celebration and relaxation.

2 drops Lavender

2 drops Juniper

2 drops Frankincense

purifying

Purifying your new home will allow you to start your new life with a fresh vitality and energy. The rejuvenating qualities of Pennyroyal will uplift, regenerate and clear the way for this new stage in your life's journey.

DO NOT USE IF PREGNANT

6 drops Pennyroyal only

clearing vibes

Your new home may carry the energies of people who have lived there before. This can be uncomfortable, particularly if some unresolved event occurred there or if the spirit of someone who died has not yet been released. In situations like this, it is best to clear out old vibes.

6 drops Juniper only

kitchen

The kitchen is one of the most important parts of your home, and the way you look after it can be a reflection of your own health and wellbeing. Wholesome organic food, lovingly prepared in a warm and inviting kitchen is the perfect recipe for nourishing both body and soul. Use these recipes to enhance the moods of your kitchen.

breezy

Create a fresh and light atmosphere for breakfast or lunch with friends and family.

2 drops Bergamot

2 drops Grapefruit

2 drops Mandarin

warming

A stimulating blend for an elegant dinner party, or that after-dinner gathering around the fireplace, sipping a fine red wine.

2 drops Black Pepper

2 drops Cinnamon

2 drops Ginger

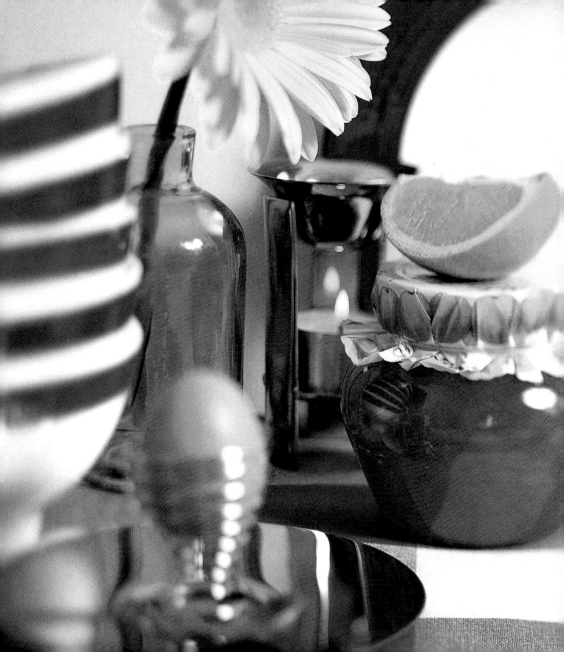

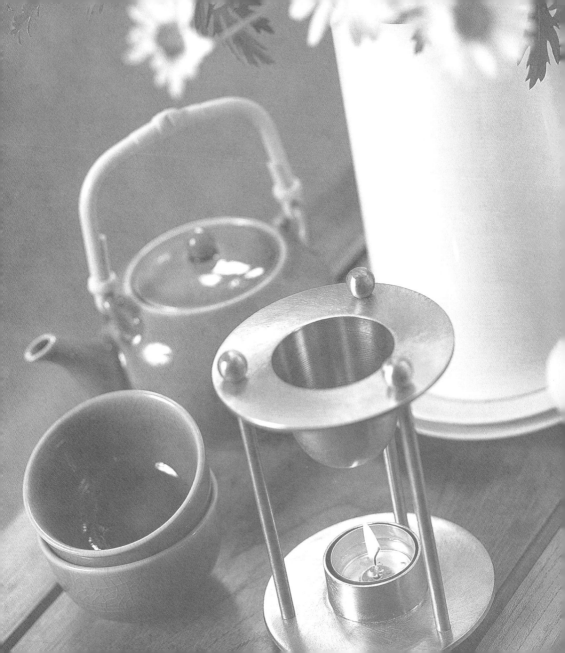

lounge/living room

Here are two ideal blends for your home's social space — the spot where friends and family gather to chat, listen to music, play games or watch movies. These mixes will evoke a sense of spirit and enchantment, and create a mood of tranquillity.

3 drops Bergamot

3 drops Geranium

or

3 drops Cinnamon

3 drops Petitgrain

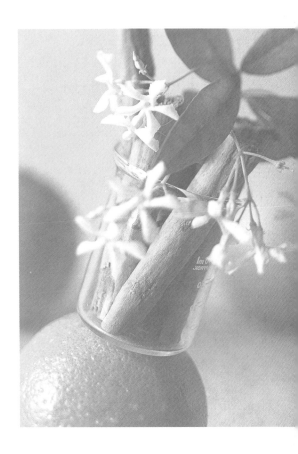

bathroom

An excellent natural alternative to common chemical air fresheners, this blend of essential oils has a fresh, clean scent without the toxic smells usually associated with chemical-based products.

1 drop Cypress
2 drops Eucalyptus
1 drop Juniper
1 drop Pine
1 drop Rosemary

toilet
For naturally eliminating any unpleasant odours.

3 drops Tea-tree
2 drops Pine
2 drops Lavender

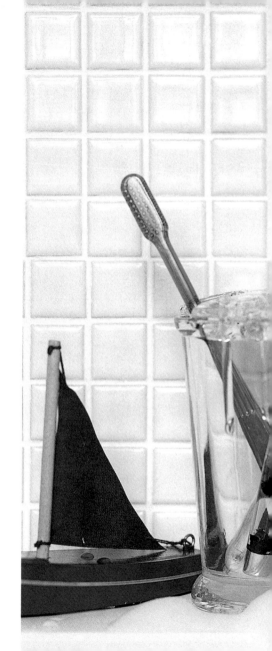

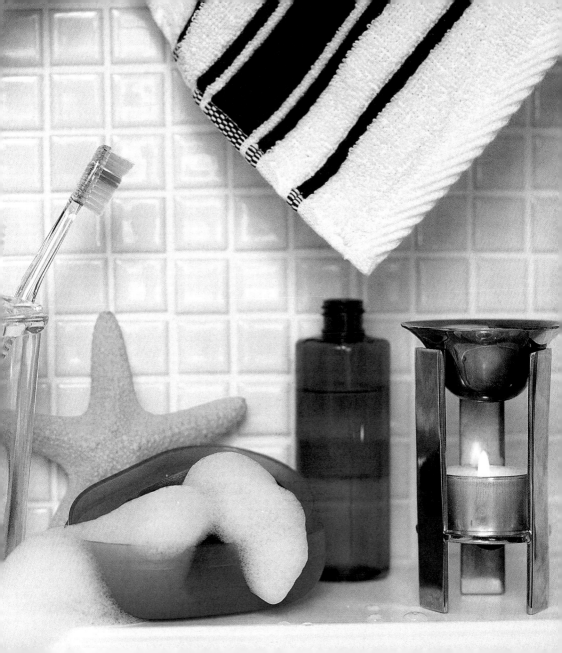

bathtime

Taking a bath gives you the time to cleanse, centre and revitalise yourself, whether you choose to be massaged by spa-jets or float in a tub. Take time out to ponder your life, pamper your body, play with your children or indulge your lover with a back scrub, a foot massage and a little heart-warming chitchat.

evening bath

This nurturing blend will encourage relaxation, help alleviate stress and tension and encourage the easy onset of a deep and rejuvenating sleep.

2 drops Geranium
2 drops Palma Rosa
2 drops Ylang Ylang
or
2 drops Ylang Ylang
2 drops Rose
2 drops Lavender

morning bath

A bracing blend to stimulate circulation and encourage the elimination of toxins, leaving you renewed, refreshed and ready to welcome the day.

2 drops Sandalwood

2 drops Cedarwood

2 drops Rosemary

or

3 drops Lime

3 drops Lavender

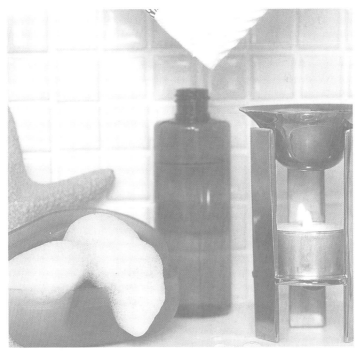

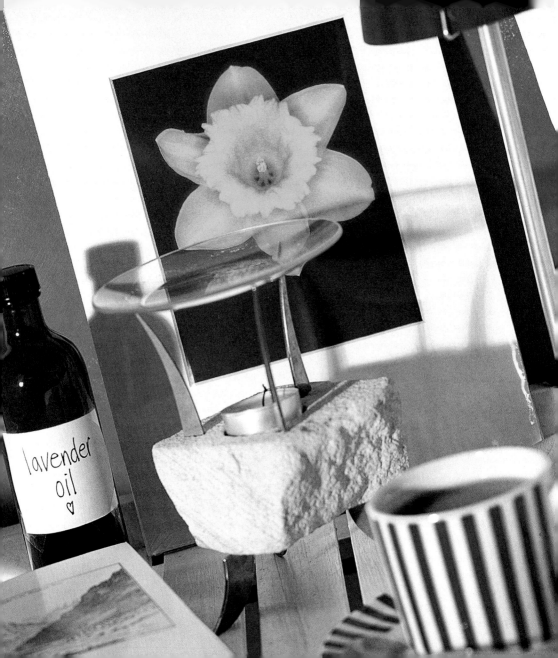

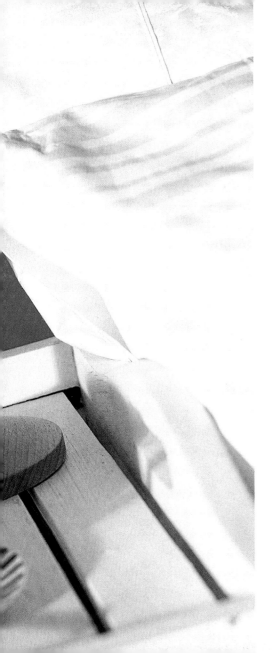

bedroom

Your bedroom can be a place of sanctuary where you retreat from the world and spend quality time by yourself. Turn your room into a peaceful, warming and inviting temple so you feel immediate comfort and ease whenever you walk in.

restful

Let this hearty yet mellow blend soothe and calm the atmosphere of your bedroom to promote restfulness and encourage a really deep sleep.

2 drops Lavender

2 drops Chamomile

2 drops Clary Sage

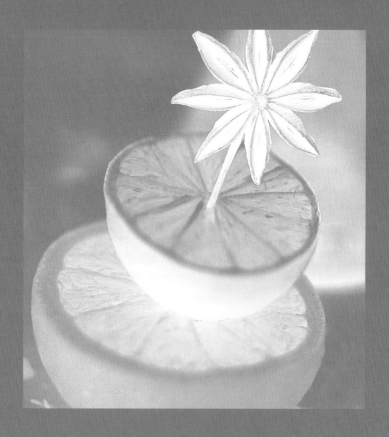

magical

Bring mystery and magic to
your bedroom. Let go of the
obvious and dive into the
mystic with this special blend.
It will evoke those special
moments of enchantment we all
carry in our hearts.

2 drops Frankincense
2 drops Patchouli
2 drops Sandalwood

masculine

Fill your bedroom with the
powerful and spirited presence
of male or 'yang' energy. A
masculine atmosphere is potent
and stimulating, vigorous,
energetic and full of warmth.

2 drops Bergamot
2 drops Lime

1 drop Cinnamon
1 drop Black Pepper
1 drop Rosemary
or
3 drops Marjoram
3 drops Cypress

feminine

The presence of feminine 'yin'
energy will bring a delicate
and healing atmosphere to
your bedroom, nourishing and
harmonising your whole body.

3 drops Bergamot
3 drops Vanilla
or
3 drops Rose Otto
2 drops Geranium
3 drops Melissa

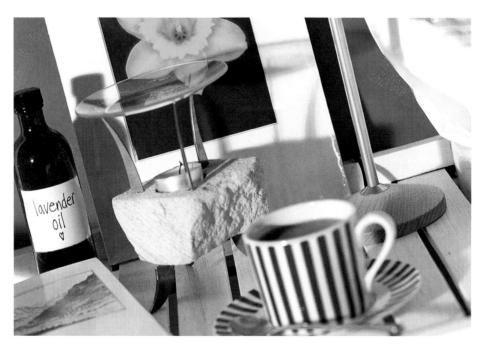

morning blend

This refreshing blend is great for beginning your day. It's definitely healthier than coffee and smells just as good! Grapefruit will really wake you up and put you in high spirits, and Rosemary and Lavender add that spark you need to be at your best at this time of day.

2 drops Grapefruit

2 drops Lavender

2 drops Rosemary

or

3 drops Orange

3 drops Rosemary

evening blend

A lovely blend to burn as the sun goes down. Ideal for bidding farewell to the day and introducing a deliciously warm and sensuous atmosphere in which to unwind and prepare for the evening's activities.

3 drops Orange

3 drops Cinnamon

or

2 drops Rosemary

2 drops Clary Sage

2 drops Geranium

oriental

Create an atmosphere of Asia in your home with the sweet and spicy fragrances of the Orient. The best way to replicate the extraordinarily unique scent of the East is to burn the essential oils in a base of orange flower water instead of plain water.

chinese

6 drops Melissa in orange flower water

japanese

6 drops Grapefruit in orange flower water

thai

6 drops Lemongrass in orange flower water

citrus

Let the uplifting tang of citrus fruits spread a happy, zesty atmosphere throughout your home. This great blend is reminiscent of a fruit tingle on a hot summer's day!

2 drops Lime

1 drop Lemongrass

1 drop Mandarin

1 drop Orange

resolving tension

Your home is your temple, your personal sanctuary. If your space is disturbed by tensions, use these blends to help resolve the problems and restore your home's peaceful atmosphere.

3 drops Juniper

3 drops Lavender

uplifting

Refresh and invigorate everyone's spirits. These oils will spark an extra burst of life energy, filling the air with a deliciously rejuvenating bouquet everyone is certain to enjoy.

2 drops Bergamot

2 drops Grapefruit

1 drop Orange

1 drop Frankincense

communicating

This recipe promotes communication and honesty. It will help to clear the air and encourage feelings of openness and closeness. These oils are known to steady and balance the emotions, awaken higher levels of being, and give you the strength and confidence to communicate successfully, without self-doubt.

3 drops Lavender
3 drops Frankincense

odours

Clear your home of unwanted smells, like stale cigarette smoke.

6 drops Juniper
or
6 drops Basil

outdoors

A pleasing and invigorating aroma for any outdoor setting, whether you're hanging out in the backyard or sitting on a balcony enjoying the cool evening air. This blend also helps to keep insects away!

2 drops Citronella
2 drops Lemongrass
2 drops Peppermint
1 drop Lavender

air fresheners

These blends will infuse your home and work environments with new aromas. Helping to clear out old odours and auras, they support the celebration of seasonal transitions.

spring and summer

Reflect on the end of winter and soak up the warmth of the beautiful sun.

spring

3 drops Melissa

3 drops Grapefruit

or

3 drops Mandarin

3 drops Black Pepper

summer

3 drops Lemon

3 drops Bergamot

or

3 drops Pine

3 drops Cypress

autumn and winter

Reflect on the passing of summer and awaken to the energising freshness of cool winds and billowing clouds.

autumn

3 drops Cedarwood

3 drops Petitgrain

or

3 drops Sandalwood

3 drops Lavender

winter

3 drops Clove

3 drops Ginger

or

3 drops Cinnamon

3 drops Orange

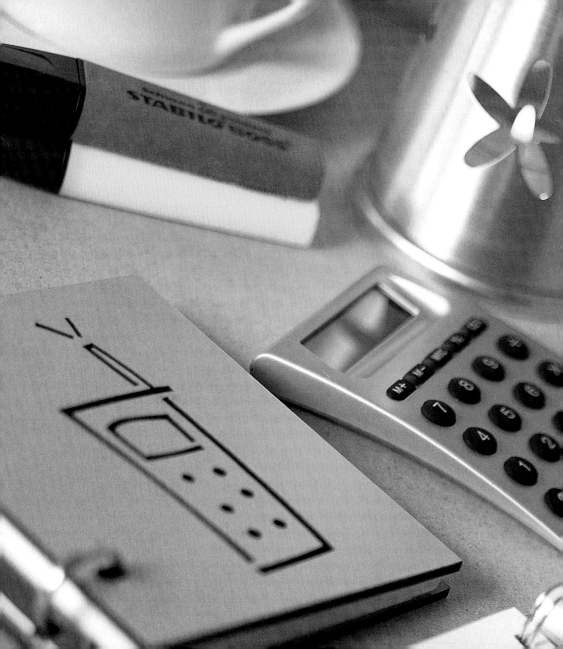

work & study

Alone, silently

the bamboo shoot

becomes a bamboo

Santoka

Most of us spend so much of our life working or studying that it's really important to make this time as relaxing and enjoyable as possible. Choose a work or study situation that nourishes your spirit as well as generates the income you need to live the life you want. Value your time at work and your input — for example, whenever you complete a task congratulate yourself on a job well done. Use the recipes following to enhance your time at work and help you make the most of your skills and capabilities.

re-energising

This is a great blend to prepare in large quantities for taking to work. These oils are known to stimulate and will help generate the extra energy we often need at low points during the day, like that mid-afternoon slump. A healthier solution than coffee or chocolate!

1 drop Lavender
2 drops Geranium
1 drop Cedarwood
2 drops Peppermint
or
2 drops Nutmeg
2 drops Rosemary
2 drops Thyme

clarity of thought

Reduce the strain on an overloaded brain. These oils will stimulate and uplift, leaving you feeling rejuvenated and newly productive.

3 drops Fennel

3 drops Lemon

or

3 drops Cardamon

3 drops Sandalwood

tension

Burn this blend to help engender feelings of inner peace and detachment. Breathe deeply, acknowledge your tensions and try to let them go with each breath you exhale. Then you will be able to see, with clarity, the reason for your tension and resolve it.

3 drops Lavender

3 drops Marjoram

frustration

If you are feeling frustrated at work, try not to react immediately to the situation or the person. Acknowledge that the frustration or tension you feel is your own. Arrange an appropriate time to talk it over with your colleague rather than let it build up and fester inside you.

2 drops Cypress
2 drops Petitgrain
2 drops Bergamot
or
2 drops Lemon
4 drops Coriander

computer fatigue

If you work long hours at a computer, make sure you do plenty of eye and body exercises to prevent any long-term harm. Insist on a good chair and make sure the computer screen is set at a comfortable eye level. These blends will help to relieve fatigue, promote stamina and re-charge your energy levels.

2 drops Basil
2 drops Lemon
2 drops Rosemary
or
1 drop Cypress
1 drop Cedarwood
1 drop Pine
2 drops Lemon

challenges

There are times when you need to challenge yourself at work, and there are times when your health is not up to par and you really need to push yourself to change your lifestyle. Whatever the challenge, these oils help to stimulate the will and the vigour to deal with anything that lies ahead.

3 drops Palma Rosa

3 drops Ginger

or

3 drops Nutmeg

3 drops Orange

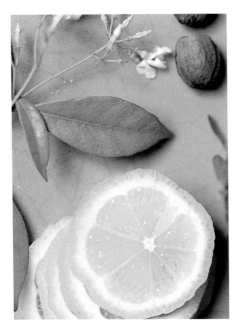

business meeting

To help facilitate the outcome of a business meeting, burn these blends approximately one hour before the meeting so the aroma has time to fill the room. At the same time, focus or meditate on your intentions for the meeting, so that your participation is clear, powerful and effective.

3 drops Cedarwood

2 drops Rosemary

2 drops Petitgrain

or

2 drops Spearmint

2 drops Lime

2 drops Lemongrass

job interview

An important moment in your life! If you really want this job, set aside some time a few days before the interview to practise how you're going to handle yourself. Answer out loud the questions you think you will be asked. For example, 'Why do you want this job?' or 'What do you think you can offer this organisation?' As you're preparing for the interview, burn one of these blends.

masculine

3 drops Peppermint

3 drops Cedarwood

or

feminine

3 drops Orange

2 drops Geranium

special events

The celebration of a store opening, a product launch or a similar special event can be enhanced by the added touch of aromatherapy. These two blends will spice up any business-social affair.

3 drops Melissa

2 drops Lemongrass

1 drop Tea-tree

or

3 drops Lime

3 drops Sandalwood

studying

The essential oils used in this recipe are known to stimulate the mind and provide clarity of thought. When studying for an exam or preparing for a presentation, use this mix to inspire and uplift you and to enhance your capacity to absorb and assimilate information.

3 drops Rosemary

2 drops Lemongrass

1 drop Basil

after work
or study

If you're the workaholic type
you may need to use a variety
of different methods to centre
and relax yourself when you
come home after a day at
work, school or university.
Meditation, yoga or a simple
walk on the beach can work
wonders. And this blend
can help.

3 drops Juniper
3 drops Melissa

stress

Stress symptoms like anxiety,
headaches or frustration are a
sign that your body is out of
balance and you need a rest.
At times like this it is vital to
rebalance your energy. Start
by changing to a healthier and
calmer lifestyle. Avoid any
stimulants while you are
moving your body from
chaos to centredness. These
soothing blends will help.

3 drops Patchouli
3 drops Vetiver
or
2 drops Petitgrain
2 drops Bergamot
2 drops Rosemary

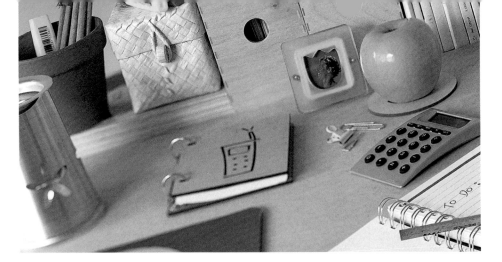

stage fright

Do you become a nervous wreck before you have to make a speech or perform before a group of people? These oils will stimulate your innate confidence to help you to find the words you want quickly and easily.

3 drops Black Pepper

3 drops Rosemary

mental fatigue

Practising a relaxation technique is the ideal way to alleviate mental fatigue, soothe your spirit and give your mind a break from day-to-day life. In your quest for a deep state of mental relaxation, these oils can help.

3 drops Rosemary

3 drops Marjoram

or

6 drops Peppermint

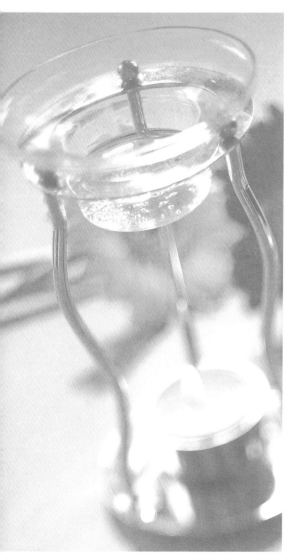

creativity

Some great blends for those times when you're feeling uninspired and need help in contacting the pure creative energy that resides within you. As well as burning these essential oils, a period of deep relaxation or a long, brisk walk will help to clear your head, boost your energy and send your inspiration soaring.

stimulating

These oils promote clarity of mind and spark the kind of sharp alertness that assists you in creating anything you want.

3 drops Mandarin

3 drops Black Pepper

focusing

These oils are traditionally known to help improve concentration and clear the mind of distractions. Uplifting and clarifying, they are an excellent support in generating feelings of confidence, conviction and capability.

3 drops Rosemary

3 drops Sage

creative visualisation

Special blends like those below can help connect you with your inner creative force. To activate this inner power, spend time alone in silence — daily if you can — and give yourself the appreciation and confidence you deserve.

2 drops Coriander

2 drops Bergamot

2 drops Neroli

or

2 drops Mandarin

2 drops Ginger

2 drops Frankincense

mind & spirit

Morning glories –

blown to the earth

and blooming again

Issa

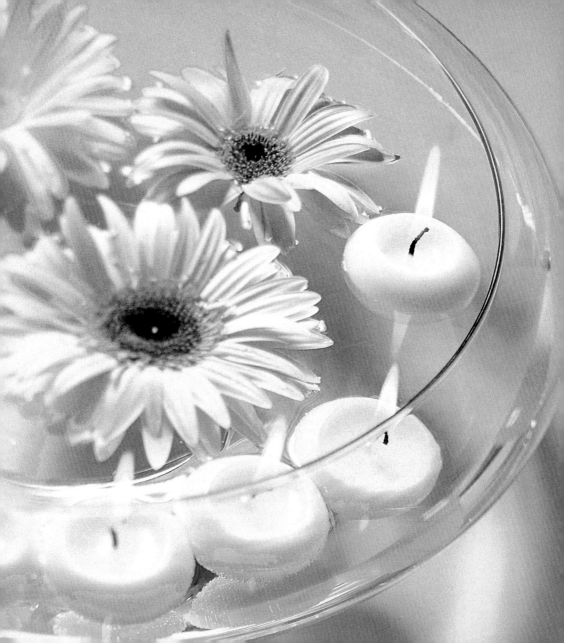

There are many ways to keep your mind and spirit strong and nourished and to enjoy your life. Treat yourself with respect. Learn to love and trust yourself. Ensure that your health is good. Follow your heart. Learn to give and receive love. Life is made up of peaks of joy and realisation and valleys of sadness and confusion. The blends in this section will help you create a life of peace and stability, passion, freedom and fulfilment — the sort of life we all deserve.

achievement

Make full use of your potential and turn your dreams and aspirations into reality. The strengthening and sharpening properties of these oils will generate feelings of clarity and decisiveness so you can celebrate what you have already achieved in life, and look forward to the challenges still to come.

2 drops Basil

2 drops Nutmeg

2 drops Sage

or

2 drops Clove

2 drops Fennel

2 drops Thyme

alertness

These uplifting oils will help sharpen your mind and eliminate fatigue. They encourage feelings of awareness and clarity of thought — a great help in seeing things clearly and making better decisions.

3 drops Angelica
3 drops Patchouli
or
3 drops Coriander
3 drops Jasmine

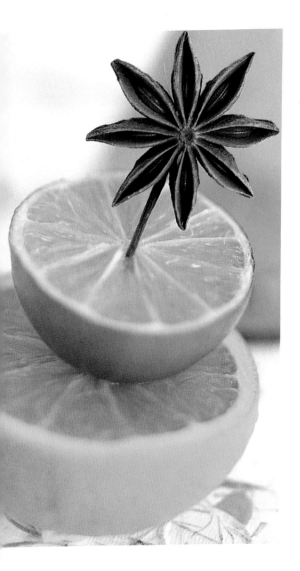

anger

In an ideal world, we need not feel any anger towards our family, friends, lovers or children. Anger can reflect our limitations, our inability to understand and see the bigger picture. These lovely aromas are for releasing deep-felt tensions and aggressions. They will create a more joyful atmosphere and induce calmness.

3 drops Grapefruit
3 drops Melissa
or
3 drops Cedarwood
3 drops Vetiver

anxiety

Burn these aromatic blends whenever you feel apprehensive or concerned about something. Their calming properties will help settle your emotions in times of distress. Maintaining a healthy lifestyle can also help to relieve anxiety, as will keeping a positive outlook. Remember that you are a capable and competent person.

3 drops Cardamon

3 drops Sandalwood

or

3 drops Patchouli

3 drops Vetiver

or

2 drops Petitgrain

2 drops Bergamot

2 drops Rosemary

apathy

These recipes will stimulate you to action at times when your energy and motivation is low. Their uplifting and refreshing aromas are great to burn at home or in the office. Including more variety in your life and increasing physical activities can also help to rejuvenate your appetite for life.

2 drops Orange

2 drops Lemon

2 drops Lime

or

3 drops Black Pepper

3 drops Grapefruit

aspiration

Make full use of your potential and achieve some of your greatest aspirations by burning these blends and contemplating what really drives and excites you. Realise what lights your inner fire then plan a way of living your dream.

2 drops Basil

2 drops Sage

2 drops Nutmeg

or

2 drops Clove

2 drops Fennel

2 drops Thyme

awareness

Awareness is a truly blissful state — a taste of eternity that comes with living totally in the moment. Spending regular time alone will help you to connect with yourself and your surroundings. Burn these blends during your times of silence and relaxation to help bring you into touch with your true being.

3 drops Juniper

3 drops Lavender

or

3 drops Lemongrass

3 drops Clary Sage

balance

Learn to appreciate the beauty and serenity of being in balance. If you have an extreme or activity-filled lifestyle, it is particularly important to incorporate some calming activities into your daily routine. Good food and relaxation exercises will help you get in touch with your inner space. These oils will create a calm and liberating atmosphere in which you can realign your energy.

6 drops Peppermint

or

6 drops Lavender

bliss

The state of bliss is when the simple things in life come alive with magic, where nature and friendship override the importance of money and a career. To evoke this enchanted state of appreciation, include joyful activities in your life, like meditation, spending time in nature, and doing fun, playful things that make you laugh. These blends will help to induce blissful feelings.

3 drops Neroli

3 drops Vanilla

or

3 drops Rose

3 drops Sandalwood

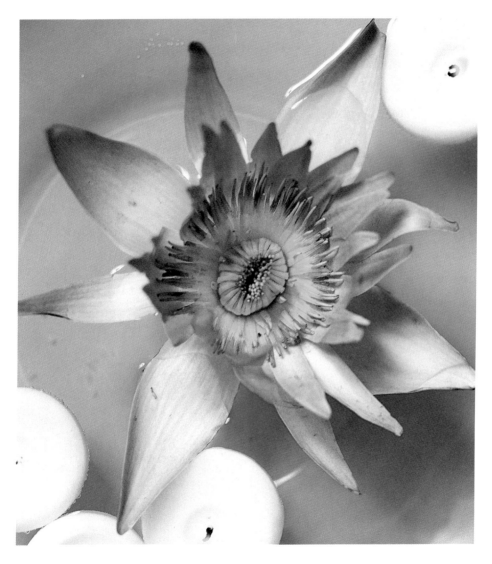

boredom

These relaxing but stimulating blends will help to relieve that feeling of being bored silly. Even though it's sometimes good to just relax and enjoy the feeling of having absolutely nothing to do, too much boredom can become unhealthy. If you find you are uninspired by your job or your life in general, pick yourself up and make some changes. Everything will flow more easily when you feel stimulated and inspired.

2 drops Peppermint

2 drops Pine

2 drops Sandalwood

or

3 drops Black Pepper

3 drops Patchouli

burn-out

When you need time out from the craziness and chaos of day-to-day life, find a nice quiet place where your spirit can rest and fill the air with these aromas. Spend some time in nature and let the smells of the bush or the beach envelop you. Nature is the ultimate healer and regenerator, and you will come back to your life feeling deeply relaxed and more alive.

3 drops Cardamon

3 drops Cedarwood

or

3 drops Coriander

3 drops Jasmine

centredness

To be centred is to be in the moment, in a space where your mind, body and soul embrace the eternal. Today's lifestyle can be stressful and confusing so staying strong and centred can be hard work. Still, to sustain your energy it is vital to remain balanced. Burn this blend and take time alone each day to really get in touch with yourself.

3 drops Hyssop
3 drops Juniper
or
3 drops Cypress
3 drops Lime

change

When you and your circumstances begin to change, realise that you are truly on the verge of flowering. Variety in life brings many lessons from which we can learn and develop; and include both negative and positive experiences. The key is to recognise change, and then, from this point of acknowledgement, to expand and mature. Burn these blends to reflect on and come to grips with these changes; they will give you the confidence to help understand where they can lead.

3 drops Grapefruit
3 drops Melissa

chill out

Take time out from emotions like worry, fear and stress and burn these blends, formulated to create a relaxing and soothing aroma to rest your whole being. They also carry qualities to lift depression and fatigue and purify the air, so you can clear your mind of any sluggish or stuck energy.

3 drops Mandarin
3 drops Lemongrass
or
3 drops Palma Rosa
3 drops Cedarwood

communication

An optimistic outlook and positive affirmations can assist in building your confidence so you can communicate clearly. Break out and undertake new endeavours to spice up your interest in life and new relationships. Burn these aromatic blends when you feel you need that extra lift to communicate.

2 drops Clove

2 drops Rosemary

2 drops Orange

or

3 drops Lavender

3 drops Frankincense

relaxed communication

Lift your confidence and increase your communication skills with this blend.

2 drops Lime

2 drops Lemon

2 drops Petitgrain

communication during transitional times

Burn the clarifying scent of cypress during periods of transition, when it's important to be calm and grounded as you seek to resolve problems of expression.

6 drops Cypress

competition

This blend has qualities that are renowned for clearing the mind, aiding the memory and grounding the body. They are perfect to burn before you face a competition or a physical and/or emotional challenge. Their calming and comforting qualities will also help you relax so you are prepared to enjoy the competition.

3 drops Chamomile
3 drops Ginger

conflict

Conflict can be a positive way to learn about yourself and others. These blends carry harmonising properties that can help spur you on to resolve conflict situations and dissolve any anxious or frustrated feelings.

3 drops Vetiver
3 drops Rosewood
or
3 drops Patchouli
3 drops Ylang Ylang

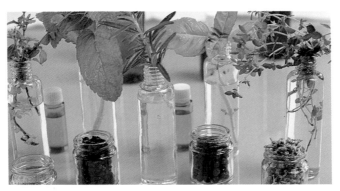

coordination

A stressful lifestyle can result in loss of precision in your movements. You may find yourself bumping into things or dropping things, or just feeling a general lack of energy and focus. These blends are for burning when you want to bring yourself back into awareness, back into the moment. They will help disperse nervousness and fatigue so you will feel much more grounded in your energy.

3 drops Rosemary

3 drops Bergamot

or

2 drops Marjoram

3 drops Thyme

1 drop Peppermint

courage

Having the will and drive to live your life at your fullest potential sometimes requires risk-taking and bravery. When your chi energy is strong you can take on life's experiences at full charge. There are many ways to increase your chi including oriental exercises such as Qigong and martial arts. These blends will fill the air with revitalising and uplifting aromas to inspire your courage.

3 drops Juniper

3 drops Cedarwood

or

3 drops Orange

3 drops Lemongrass

depression

Unresolved experiences can express themselves in emotions like sadness, fear and anger and can sometimes evolve into depression. The stabilising qualities of these blends can promote feelings of joy and tranquillity. Burn them while you consider ways to pull yourself out of the depression cycle.

3 drops Bergamot

3 drops Grapefruit

or

2 drops Basil

2 drops Vetiver

2 drops Neroli

sedative blend

This blend will help to break the tormenting cycle of thoughts that often accompanies depression.

2 drops Chamomile

2 drops Clary Sage

1 drop Lavender

1 drop Sandalwood

non-sedative blend

A stimulating, uplifting blend to alleviate the feelings of torpidity and despondency that are symptomatic of depression.

2 drops Bergamot

2 drops Geranium

2 drops Melissa

or

2 drops Sandalwood

2 drops Ylang Ylang

2 drops Orange

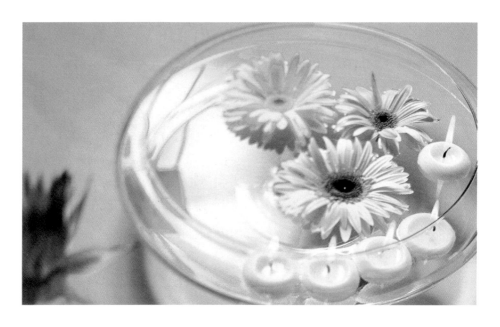

emotional healing

Sometimes emotional wounds can affect us just as much as physical ones. Burn these blends when you are feeling hurt and let their soothing and uplifting qualities comfort you.

3 drops Peppermint

3 drops Cedarwood

or

3 drops Geranium

3 drops Lavender

or

2 drops Mandarin

2 drops Lavender

2 drops Patchouli

excitability

These blends circulate calming aromas and will help soothe overactive emotions. Burn these blends in your bedroom, light a candle and play your favourite relaxing music. Spend twenty minutes doing this every evening and you will experience renewed calmness and joy.

2 drops Melissa

2 drops Neroli

2 drops Ylang Ylang

or

2 drops Juniper

2 drops Clary Sage

2 drops Chamomile

exhaustion

After a hard day at work, use these blends to help ease your fatigue and increase your energy. Combine them with a good night's sleep and awake feeling renewed and positive about the coming day. If you constantly feel exhausted you may need to reconsider your lifestyle. Take time out to nurture your body with plenty of exercise and rest.

2 drops Peppermint

2 drops Lemon

2 drops Lime

or

2 drops Rosemary

2 drops Basil

2 drops Thyme

envy

Being envious can make you feel really uncomfortable. Try to understand what it is about a particular person that makes you envious. It may be that you admire qualities in them that you know you have inside yourself but are not expressing. Take this feeling of envy as an opportunity to learn more about yourself. You may find that eventually your envy turns to admiration and friendship.

2 drops Cypress
2 drops Basil
2 drops Pennyroyal (NOT WHEN PREGNANT)
or
3 drops Rose
3 drops Melissa

fear

Fear is an indication of low 'chi' energy that can really hinder you in experiencing the full magic of life. Try not to hide your fear behind security symbols. Instead, look inside to see where the fear first began and try to resolve the event that triggered it initially. Burn these blends to help resolve the fear and fill your life with joy and wellbeing.

3 drops Bergamot
2 drops Lavender
1 drop Basil
or
3 drops Basil
3 drops Geranium

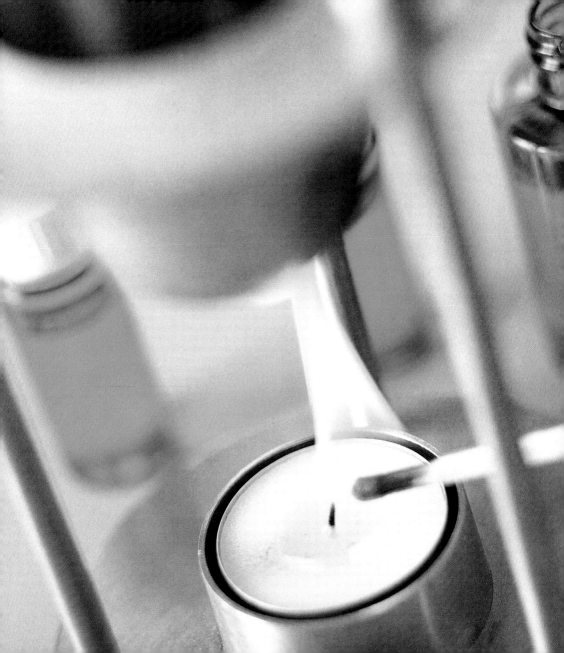

focus

Burn these powerful blends when you need extra courage and energy to really focus on and achieve what you want in your life. These aromas are known for their calming qualities, and are strengthening in times of confusion or hardship. They will help you to centre yourself so you can fully tap into your own potential.

3 drops Frankincense
3 drops Rosewood
or
6 drops Myrrh

grief

These oils are known for their comforting qualities and will help you cope with the sadness, upheaval and depression caused by grief and shock. Burning them during such deep and intense times will assist you in letting go and expressing your grief.

2 drops Basil
2 drops Vetiver
2 drops Neroli
or
2 drops Marjoram
2 drops Melissa
2 drops Bergamot
or
3 drops Palma Rosa
3 drops Grapefruit

guilt

Guilt can be more damaging than the actual act that provoked it. Living your own truth and following your intuition will lessen any guilty feelings. Burning this blend will help disperse anxious thoughts and induce a more uplifting and conscience-clearing mood.

2 drops Cypress

2 drops Pine

2 drops Lemon

guilt from the past

If you are aware that you are stuck in past experiences, also understand that unresolved emotions may cause problems in later life. Search for healing ways to let go of your guilt, such as learning to forgive and understand yourself. Try to identify the positive outcomes from these past experiences.

2 drops Patchouli

2 drops Geranium

2 drops Ginger

harmony

To really use your own energy to the best of your ability is easier when you have an understanding of your body's level of balance. Help yourself to achieve harmony in the best way you can. If you live in a stressed state, balance this with relaxing activities. If you lead an extreme lifestyle, balance this out with a diet that keeps you strong and healthy, and get regular massages and exercise. Burn these oils to create a soft, still atmosphere so you can appreciate the true beauty of existence.

3 drops Mandarin
3 drops Orange

healing

Life is a journey along a river of learning and discovery and one of its greatest experiences is learning to heal ourselves. Many of us are looking for ways to help resolve our problems and heal emotional wounds. These blends will warm and comfort you, and uplift your spirits during the healing process.

2 drops Lavender
2 drops Mandarin
2 drops Patchouli
or
3 drops Peppermint
3 drops Cedarwood
or
3 drops Geranium
3 drops Lavender

impatience

Lack of patience may indicate poor health and can be a sign that you need to take better care of yourself. Burn this blend and carry out some soul-soothing exercises to help relieve your impatience and irritability and put you in touch with the lighter side of life again.

2 drops Lavender
2 drops Valerian
1 drop Bergamot
1 drop Clary Sage
or
3 drops Marjoram
3 drops Chamomile
or
3 drops Melissa
3 drops Lime

indecision

If you really want to make the right choices in life, rebalance your energies first to avoid making rash decisions. Exercise or meditation can help to get you out of your head and into your body so your heart can tell you which is the right path to take. These blends will help you focus your thoughts and feelings to get to the heart of what you really want.

3 drops Cedarwood
3 drops Melissa
or
3 drops Melissa
3 drops Mandarin

inspiration

Feeling inspired makes your spirits soar. When you are in good health and in tune with yourself and the universe, wonderful opportunities and positive situations will come your way. Whether you are searching for inspiration in your work, study or artistic life, looking to generate cash or just to rearrange your furniture, these stimulating oils will help to clear the air. They will give you a lift and create space for the joy of real inspiration to enter your life.

3 drops Basil
3 drops Geranium
or
3 drops Fennel
3 drops Lime

joy

We are all creators of our own lives and masters of bringing ourselves fulfilment and joy. Each day we make choices that affect our future, whether it be eating well to preserve our health or following our hearts intuitively so our energy can carry us along the right path. Appreciate the gift you have right now — the present moment. These oils are known to uplift the spirits and will bring you feelings of optimism and euphoria.

6 drops Neroli
or
6 drops Rose
or
6 drops Jasmine

laughter

We all need to have more fun in life and sometimes laugh at the chaos all around us. Learning how to take time out from being serious is a definite way to enrich your soul. These delicious aromas bring a warm, freeing vibe to a room, and their positive and stimulating qualities will enhance liveliness, joy and spontaneity — all of which spark laughter.

3 drops Ginger
3 drops Grapefruit
or
3 drops Lime
3 drops Petitgrain

letting go

These blends will help give you the initiative to gently detach yourself from people or events that you feel you need to let go. Widely used for dispelling grief, loneliness, fear and anxiety, this is an infusion to burn as you intelligently consider the circumstance you are in. They will provide the inner warmth and support you need to move on.

3 drops Marjoram
3 drops Calendula
or
3 drops Melissa
3 drops Grapefruit
or
3 drops Cedarwood
3 drops Geranium

loneliness

Loneliness is a difficult emotion; it can bring up feelings of sadness and anger. Burn these blends and spend time thinking about yourself, about your direction, and what you can do to attract the right people into your life. Repeated loneliness may be a sign that you are not really living your truth, and/or that you are not living in the right environment, one where you can truly blossom.

3 drops Lemon Verbena

3 drops Ylang Ylang

or

2 drops Rosemary

2 drops Lavender

2 drops Ylang Ylang

loss of appetite

This is a sign that some aspect of your health is off-centre or that you are in a transitory phase. Loss of appetite can also mean a loss of will or a lack of direction in life. Burn these blends while reflecting on why your appetite has diminished and what is needed to revive it. If the situation persists, consult a health professional.

3 drops Fennel

3 drops Geranium

or

3 drops Fennel

3 drops Sandalwood

moving on

It's always an exciting time when you relinquish the old and move forward with renewed energy and a sense of confidence. These blends will give you an extra charge to keep you focused on your new path.

3 drops Petitgrain
3 drops Cypress
or
3 drops Chamomile
3 drops Frankincense

nervous tension

Burn these essential oils to help you relax when you are feeling uneasy, nervous and vulnerable. Known for their settling and sedative qualities, they will help take the edge off feelings of strain and pressure, and encourage rest and tranquillity.

3 drops Patchouli
3 drops Vetiver
or
3 drops Melissa
3 drops Bergamot

oppression

Feeling weighed down lately, as if everything is too much effort? If things get too much and you feel heavy and depressed, think back to how it feels to be calm and allow the heavy oppressive energy to flow through you and out of you. Burn these blends to create a tranquil atmosphere in which mind and body can relax and you can enjoy some well-deserved peace.

2 drops Lemon
2 drops Bergamot
1 drop Petitgrain
1 drop Geranium
or
3 drops Rosemary
3 drops Peppermint

passion

Passion flies straight from the heart with no stops or detours. Feeling passionate about life, your lover, your family, your friends and yourself is the ultimate involvement. Discovering your own passion is easier when you are balanced and living your truth without inhibition. Release yourself into your passion and let your life ignite.

3 drops Rosewood
3 drops Vetiver
or
3 drops Ginger
3 drops Geranium

peace

A peaceful world is possible!
You can help by starting with
finding your own inner peace.
Your serenity will have a positive
effect on everyone around you.
If we all love and support each
other, we can all live together
in peace and harmony on this
beautiful planet.

3 drops Sandalwood
3 drops Bergamot
or
3 drops Palma Rosa
3 drops Mandarin

prayer

For this private ritual, find a
quiet place that is sacred to you
and use these blends to create
an atmosphere of peace and
reflection. Prayer is a time for
insight into those profound life
questions, as well as a means
of self-affirmation.

3 drops Frankincense
3 drops Myrrh
or
3 drops Sandalwood
3 drops Geranium

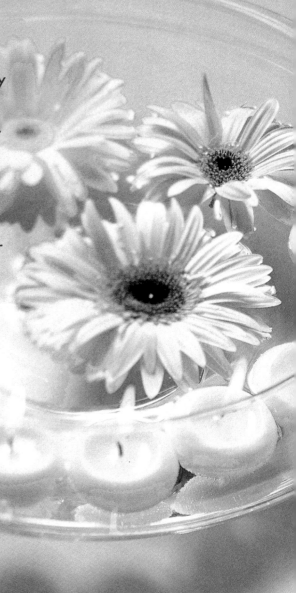

rebalancing

One way to sustain your energy in life is to introduce balancing qualities into your daily routine. Trying to keep our sensitive selves strong and balanced to face the ever-changing tide of events that occur day by day, season by season, year by year requires constant awareness. These oils will induce calmness and balance so you can consciously consider all the moves you are making in your life right now.

2 drops Lemon

2 drops Peppermint

2 drops Rosemary

or

3 drops Thyme

3 drops Lemon

recharging

Release past tensions and find the drive and motivation to recharge your batteries and move ahead. These stimulating blends will surround you with feelings of strength during this time of change. Take the time to do spirit-enlivening activities to keep your energy levels moving.

3 drops Mandarin
3 drops Black Pepper
or
3 drops Ginger
3 drops Lemon

relaxation

Being relaxed can be about surrendering your whole self to the flow of life — allowing your being to experience life's ups, downs and plateaus. These blends carry soothing and nurturing qualities and will help release tension, fear and agitation. They will induce feelings of calm and promote restful sleep. Ideal to burn when you feel uptight or just need to unwind after a long day.

 3 drops Lavender
3 drops Chamomile
or
3 drops Marjoram
3 drops Thyme

resolution

The balancing and vibrant aromas of this powerful blend create a cheerful and uplifting atmosphere to strengthen your purpose in life. Writing down your resolutions and reading them anew each morning is a great way to remain strong.

3 drops Grapefruit

3 drops Melissa

sadness

This blend will instil a sense of calmness and acceptance about your sadness, and disperse your suffering so that you can face what is really happening. Accept that you feel sad and that this is a valid emotion. Then seek ways to transform your sadness into joy and understanding.

3 drops Bergamot

3 drops Grapefruit

or

3 drops Rosewood

3 drops Petitgrain

security

One thing we can be certain about is that life is constantly changing. Just when we think we know someone or have a grasp on a situation, it seems to change. These oils are known to stabilise and strengthen emotions and will evoke a warm, secure and reassuring atmosphere to help retain your strength and balance.

3 drops Basil

3 drops Geranium

or

3 drops Melissa

3 drops Chamomile

or

2 drops Sandalwood

2 drops Bergamot

2 drops Petitgrain

self-acknowledgement

These blends will help you to generate a sense of value and belief in yourself, and calm emotions such as jealousy, anxiety, frustration and anger. They are known for their settling qualities as well as their ability to evoke inner fire and sensuality, sparking your own sense of confidence and self-worth.

3 drops Vanilla

3 drops Ylang Ylang

or

3 drops Cedarwood

3 drops Neroli

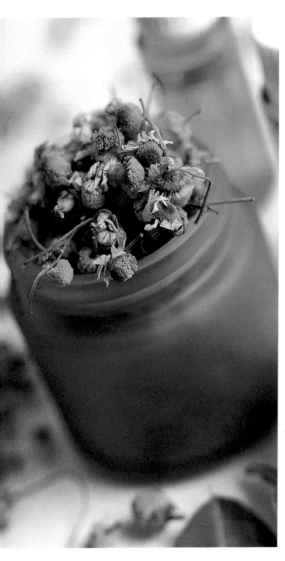

self-confidence

Self-confidence attracts positive people and situations that can bring tangible benefits to your life. Feeling centred and healthy will increase your self-confidence. Negative experiences are also part of life, so it can take a huge effort and commitment to create and sustain confidence in yourself, your work and in your relationships. Burn these blends, focus on your positive attributes, follow your heart and appreciate who you are.

3 drops Nutmeg
3 drops Orange
or
2 drops Lemongrass
2 drops Lime
2 drops Orange

self-therapy

Burn these oils during times when you are working on healing yourself and coming face to face with your hidden side. There are many ways to improve your wellbeing, the ultimate goal being to realise your unique inner essence.

6 drops Cypress

or

3 drops Basil

3 drops Lemon

serenity

Try to capture an individual essence of serenity by spending more time close to nature, as well as more 'quality time' on your own. Learn to appreciate your stillness and harmony. Finding your own serenity is a beautiful experience. Use these oils to create a space where you can be quiet with yourself.

2 drops Ylang Ylang

2 drops Sandalwood

2 drops Valerian

or

3 drops Melissa

3 drops Chamomile

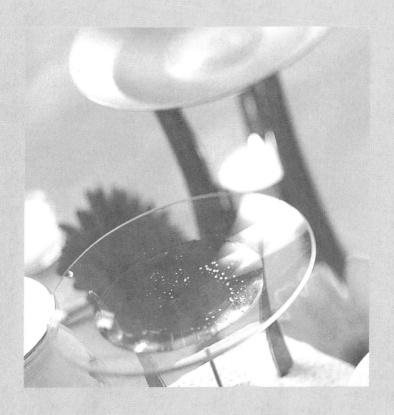

stagnation

Although we may believe we
have let go of past experiences
and relationships, our bodies
often carry these imprints
throughout our lives. Indications
we still have unresolved issues
can include lack of energy
and sexual appetite and
periods of depression. These
blends of essential oils contain
stimulating qualities to
encourage you to move
forward cleanly and happily.

2 drops Marjoram

2 drops Orange

2 drops Thyme

or

2 drops Cypress

2 drops Black Pepper

2 drops Geranium

strength

Start strengthening your spirit
today! Don't be influenced by
other people's opinions; find
your own truth. Spend time
developing and trusting your
own intuition and building your
self-esteem. Learn to be your
own best friend and recognise
your incredible inner potential.
These blends will envelop
you with warmth and security,
encouraging feelings of
confidence, positiveness
and fulfilment.

3 drops Orange

3 drops Coriander

or

2 drops Sandalwood

2 drops Ylang Ylang

2 drops Orange

suspicion

Burn these blends when you're suffering bouts of negative emotions such as suspicion and depression. These refreshing oils are known to promote clear thinking and increase mental alertness, which will help to ease feelings of inadequacy and fear.

3 drops Bergamot

3 drops Neroli

or

2 drops Pine

2 drops Cypress

2 drops Rosemary

tranquillity

To attain a state of tranquillity, your body needs to be in perfect balance. When body, mind and spirit are all healthy and flowing, we can effortlessly connect to a tranquil inner space.

3 drops Lavender

3 drops Bergamot

or

3 drops Cypress

3 drops Juniper

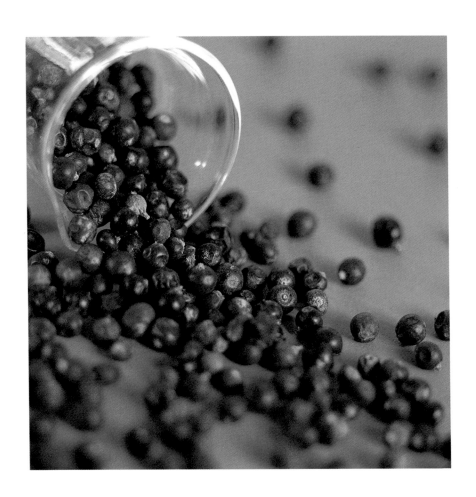

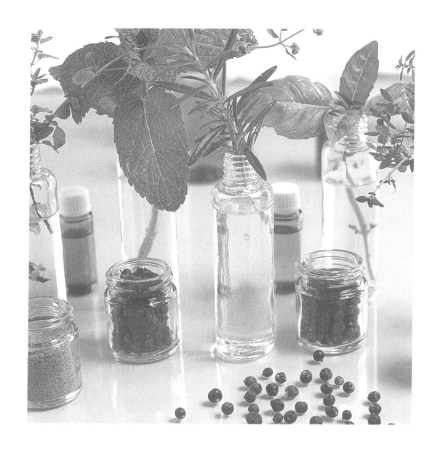

vagueness

Are you constantly vague or feel that you're somehow missing out on life? Trying to be more grounded in your everyday life can help you regain your focus and drive. These blends will assist in energising your body and clearing away the mental fatigue.

3 drops Lemon
3 drops Rosemary
or
3 drops Basil
3 drops Bergamot

weakness

The feeling of physical and spiritual weakness is similar to feeling hungry, undernourished and unfulfilled. Consider practicing some oriental discipline such as Tai Chi, Qigong or one of the martial arts to build up your 'chi' energy. These uplifting blends will promote clarity of mind while you ponder the best way to manifest to the world that dynamic person within.

2 drops Black Pepper
2 drops Clove
2 drops Fennel
or
2 drops Palma Rosa
2 drops Lavender
2 drops Grapefruit

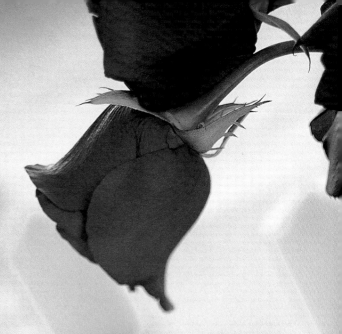

White camellias falling –

the only sound in the

moonlit evening

Ranko

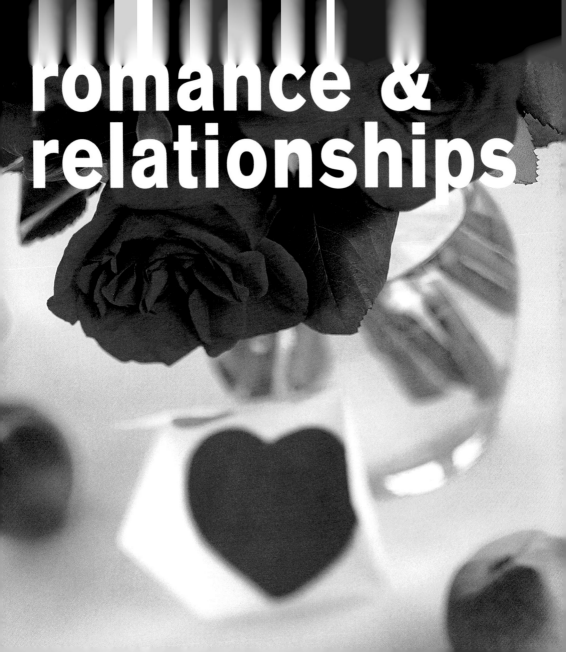

romance &
relationships

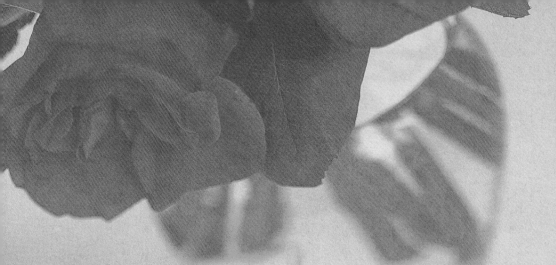

Falling in love, starting a relationship or indulging in some playful flirting can be among the more exciting moments in life, resulting in a variety of enhanced feelings. The key to intimacy with others is an open heart so you can see their beauty and appreciate that life is flowing with synchronicity. As essential oils directly influence the part of our brain which is responsible for our general behaviour, you will find that they can enhance your love life as well.

romantic dinner

Spoil your lover or partner with a specially prepared dinner. Create a little magic by lighting candles, playing music and burning one of these relaxing and warming blends.

2 drops Ylang Ylang
2 drops Vetiver
or
1 drop pure Rose oil
1 drop Sandalwood
in a Rosewater base

togetherness

Enhance closeness and celebrate the moment of merging into one. These extraordinary aromas are so special, they will leave you both feeling soft, warm and caring.

2 drops Vetiver
2 drops Rosewood
2 drops Bergamot
or
3 drops Geranium
3 drops Cinnamon

sweet sensuality

This deliciously feminine fragrance will evoke subtle sensuous and amorous sensations.

3 drops Ylang Ylang

1 drop Vanilla

1 drop Geranium

1 drop Sandalwood

Burn this blend to create a sensual atmosphere for an intimate encounter with that special person in your life.

3 drops Clary Sage

3 drops Ylang Ylang

erotic

A delicious blend with a strong yet delicate aroma to give you the confidence to express the eroticism within. Relax, put on some romantic music, soak in a tub then dress yourself in something special.
Concentrate on the physical. Enjoy every touch, every movement, every breath.

2 drops Sandalwood

3 drops Ylang Ylang

1 drop Patchouli or Rosemary

or

1 drop Petitgrain

2 drops Ylang Ylang

1 drop Geranium

1 drop Patchouli

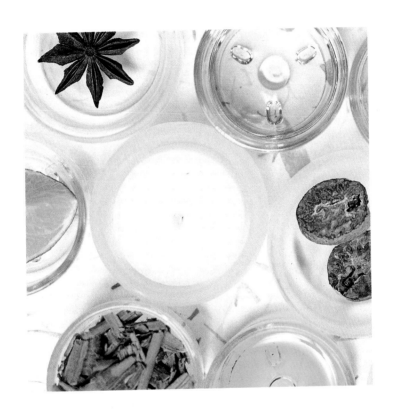

aphrodisiac

These oils are traditionally known to enhance desire and sensuality. They create a still yet expectant atmosphere that will help to open you up physically and emotionally. Their beautiful sweet aromas will evoke a warm and luxurious atmosphere.

2 drops Ylang Ylang
2 drops Clary Sage
2 drops Jasmine

slow seduction

If you want to make your lovemaking longer and more sensuous, burn this blissfully calming blend. This delicious aroma will stoke the fires of passion, helping you to relax and languidly surrender to your lover's desires.

3 drops Clary Sage
3 drops Sandalwood

sensual massage

Burn one of these strong yet subtle blends of essential oils while massaging your lover. A sensual massage can be the perfect catalyst for opening up to each other before making love. We all need physical and emotional nourishment, and massage is one of the most healing ways to let others know they are cherished.

2 drops Sandalwood
2 drops Coriander
in a Rosewater base
or
2 drops Lime
2 drops Ylang Ylang
in a Vanilla water base

sacred sex

Opening your heart and body for slow, intimate sex can take some preparation. Light candles, take a bath together, talk from the heart — whatever it takes to create a space of total togetherness so you can fully enjoy the ecstasy that comes from an exceptional union.

2 drops Vetiver
2 drops Ylang Ylang
2 drops Patchouli
or
2 drops Rose Otto
2 drops Palma Rosa
2 drops Geranium

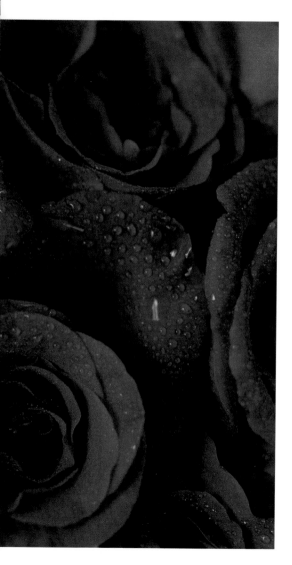

increase sex drive

To feel more confident and sexually energised, burn these blends before and during sex. These powerful and stimulating aromas will give an arousing boost with excess energy to share.

3 drops Ginger
3 drops Geranium

obsession

To help release the blocked and murky energy of obsessive feelings, burn this blend and consider where the feelings are coming from. Practise letting go of your obsession. Once you have let go, you will find an abundant world of joy and innocence awaiting you.

3 drops Neroli

3 drops Chamomile

or

6 drops Frankincense

frigidity

When you experience periods of so-called sexual inadequacy, try not to blame yourself or to think there's something wrong. Try to find out why you feel this way. These blends will help to relax you physically and promote the feelings of security and self-worth that will help you to open up again.

2 drops Neroli

2 drops Ylang Ylang

1 drop Jasmine

1 drop Rose

heartbroken

There is no easy way to heal this pain. The heart is so fragile and vulnerable, so easily wounded. Try to value your time of grieving. Don't deny your feelings or pretend to be strong — your heart will only take longer to heal. Let your tears flow and let go of the pain. This blend will help you work through this difficult time.

2 drops Bergamot

2 drops Juniper

2 drops Sandalwood

or

3 drops Patchouli

3 drops Lime

or

3 drops Basil

3 drops Orange

separation

It's always hard to leave friends, lovers and family. Whenever you're feeling sad about separation, these blends will comfort and cheer you. Sometimes spending time away from loved ones is what you need to allow your true nature to manifest itself in all its beauty.

3 drops Rosemary

3 drops Bergamot

or

3 drops Peppermint

3 drops Lemon

moving on

Although it may be painful, moving on is often the thing to do. This potion can help you through the difficult phase of letting go. This can be an important and life-transforming experience, but can also bring times of feeling downhearted and insecure. Keep to your vision and stay true to your dream.

3 drops Cypress
3 drops Lemon

celibacy

In celibate phases of your life, it is important to focus on the positive things the world has to offer. This can be a wonderful time of discovering new depths within yourself. Marjoram, with its warming and nurturing qualities, is traditionally used as a sedative. It is especially beneficial for those entering celibacy after a relationship break-up. It can help to ease the pain of physical separation and smooth the transition to new beginnings.

6 drops Marjoram

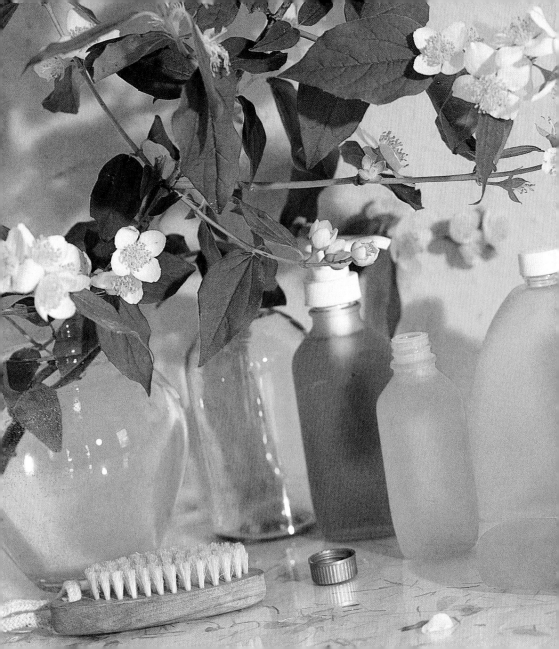

body

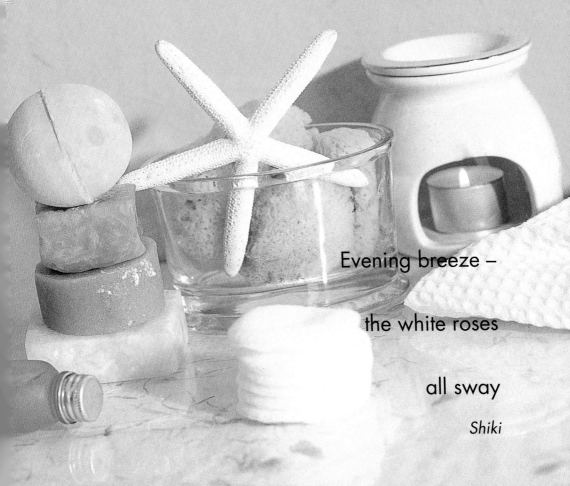

Evening breeze –

the white roses

all sway

Shiki

Your state of health can be reflected in your emotions, the way you look at yourself and others and the way you handle the different experiences of life. Physical health problems, as well as signalling the need for a change of lifestyle, can be an enlightening opportunity to learn more about yourself.

The blends in this section are to be vaporised only. They will circulate soothing and joyful aromas to help alleviate the emotions that people suffer as a result of various health conditions.

These recipes will not cure illness. It is essential to obtain professional advice when symptoms of ill-health arise.

NOTE: Do not use essential oils on your body when undertaking chemotherapy treatment.

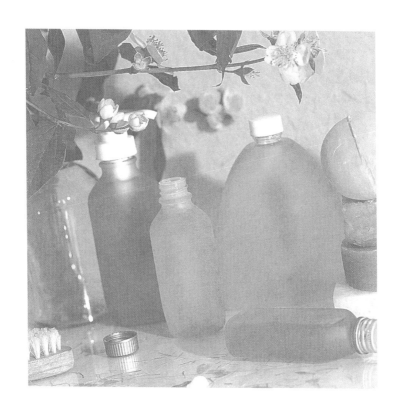

acupuncture

There are many forms of healing that help to release blockages caused by stuck emotional energy, including acupuncture, colourpuncture, Qigong, shiatsu massage and others. In acupuncture, needles are used on specific points to stimulate or impede energy and therefore release blocks to allow healing to take place.

2 drops Tea-tree
2 drops Cypress
2 drops Pine
or
3 drops Lemon
3 drops Basil

anti-viral

These refreshing essential oils are known for their medicinal, purifying and therapeutic qualities. They circulate rejuvenating and energising aromas to trigger feelings of freshness and clarity. They are the optimal blends to burn when your condition is infectious.

2 drops Neroli
2 drops Tea-tree
1 drop Eucalyptus
1 drop Thyme

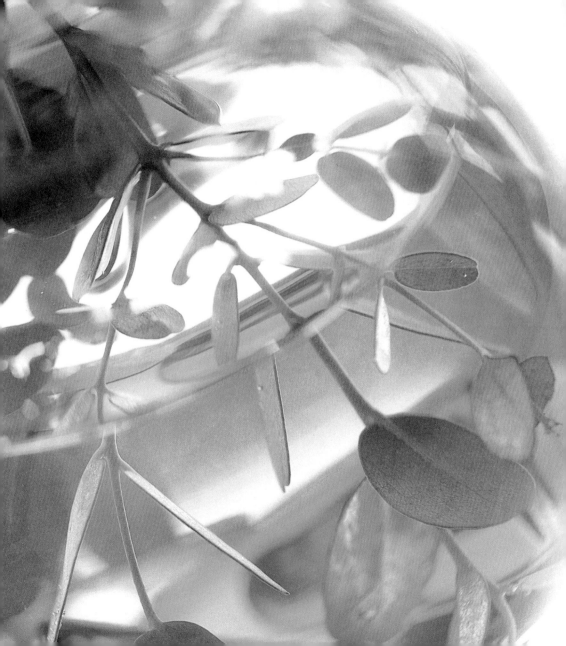

asthma

Asthma is increasingly common in Western society. Known for their comforting and rejuvenating qualities, these aromas will help strengthen emotional and physical weaknesses like fear, nervousness and anxiety, which are often associated with asthma attacks. Regular professional advice is essential.

**6 drops Frankincense
(to deepen and slow the
breathing)**
or
3 drops Thyme
3 drops Myrrh

bronchitis

These oils will help to relieve the emotional symptoms of bronchitis like depression, irritation and general low energy. Their nurturing aromas will help to promote a restful night's sleep.

3 drops Angelica
3 drops Clary Sage
or
2 drops Lavender
2 drops Bergamot
2 drops Chamomile

cleansing

When you feel the need to cleanse your body, your mind and your environment, these blends will give you the impetus to do this. Known for their uplifting and head-clearing qualities, they help improve mental alertness, and shake off confusion or lack of motivation. They are good to burn when you need to make decisions, or when you're in the process of changing your life's direction.

3 drops Cajuput

3 drops Lemon

or

3 drops Frankincense

3 drops Cardamon

fasting

A blend to keep your mind alert while you are fasting.

1 drop Lemon

1 drop Rosemary

1 drop Lemongrass

1 drop Peppermint

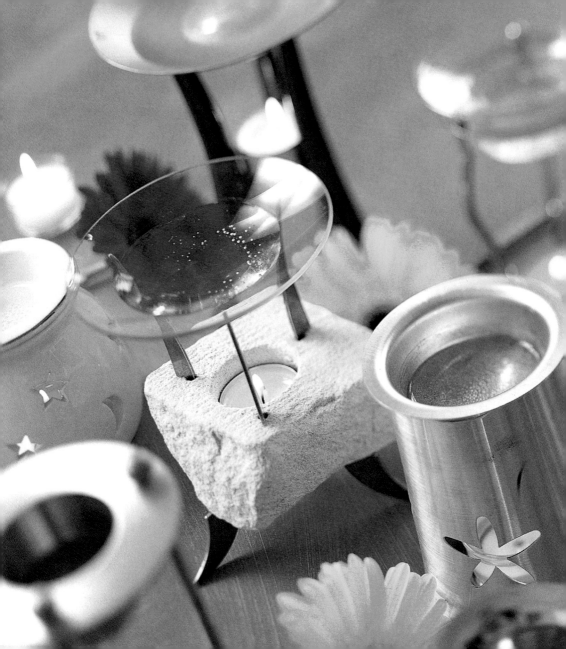

fatigue

Feeling constantly tired can be frustrating and sometimes the first sign of other health problems. These blends can help to relieve physical and mental exhaustion. They will fill the atmosphere with a refreshing, calming aroma to elevate your mood. A great remedy for tired minds that have been worrying or studying too hard.

6 drops Basil

or

3 drops Pine

3 drops Marjoram

fever

These oils work to clear and cool the head when you're feeling feverish and unwell. As well as seeking professional help, burn these blends while you allow your body to discharge unwanted toxins.

3 drops Lavender

3 drops Bergamot

or

3 drops Eucalyptus

3 drops Fennel

flu prevention

When summer turns to autumn or winter evolves into spring, your body may need to discharge toxins accumulated during the preceding season. This blend will create a warm and comforting atmosphere to keep you feeling nurtured and help to ward off any flu viruses that might be hanging around.

3 drops Clove

3 drops Cinnamon

This combination will help to clear the air:

3 drops Bergamot

3 drops Lavender

general malaise

To ease restlessness, apathy and general low energy, these blends are designed to reassure through times of transition as well as assist in releasing past heartaches and tensions. Let their aromas fill the room, to produce a nurturing and restful environment.

3 drops Chamomile

3 drops Lavender

or

3 drops Cypress

3 drops Marjoram

hangover

Too much alcohol can result in dehydration, depression, tiredness and loss of vitality. When your body is suffering the effects of excess alcohol, try to balance out this extreme yin condition with good-quality yang foods such as miso soup and bancha tea. These blends are beneficial for grounding and centring yourself when in this extreme physical state.

2 drops Ginger

2 drops Cinnamon

1 drop Sandalwood

1 drop Clove

To help alleviate the tiredness.

2 drops Grapefruit

2 drops Mandarin

2 drops Fennel

headache

These refreshing and clarifying blends will induce a warm and nurturing atmosphere for rest and rejuvenation when suffering headaches or migraine.

3 drops Lavender

3 drops Peppermint

or

3 drops Rosemary

3 drops Eucalyptus

heart palpitations

Heart palpitations or 'panic attacks' can be a frightening experience and are increasingly common today. They are often the result of long-term repressed and unresolved emotions and a sign that your body is out of balance. These blends are good to burn when you feel your heart straining. Together with special breathing techniques, these oils will help to engender calmness within.

2 drops Lavender

2 drops Melissa

1 drop Neroli

1 drop Ylang Ylang

heart strengthening

Healing your heart on a spiritual level will help it to heal physically as well. Try to dedicate twenty minutes each morning and evening to practising relaxation. Visualise yourself enveloped by a huge warm sun that is sending limitless warmth and nutrients to your heart. Do activities that keep your heart calm, avoid stimulants and open yourself to the people who really care about you.

1 drop Lavender

1 drop Marjoram

1 drop Peppermint

1 drop Rose

1 drop Rosemary

insomnia

There are many ways you can induce a good night's sleep. If you are suffering from anxiety and worry, try to calm yourself by playing relaxing music and reading a book to give yourself some uplifting affirmations. You could also try doing more exercise to disperse your energy positively. Emotional problems such as worry and depression can cause sleeping difficulties. Aromatherapy massage and yoga are highly recommended to help you relax.

2 drops Sandalwood

2 drops Juniper

2 drops Ylang Ylang

- **Add Benzoin for extra strength.**
- **Add Bergamot to relieve depression.**
- **Add Clary Sage to relieve tension.**
- **Add Marjoram to relieve loneliness.**

jet lag

One cure for jet lag is to jump into the ocean as soon as possible after landing. Salt water is extremely 'yang' and will clear away much of the 'yin' energy accumulated while flying. To encourage your body to fit in with the local time schedule, try having a massage, and doing some calming activities.
The following blends are created to help you relax so you can sleep at the desired time.

morning arrival
2 drops Lavender

2 drops Grapefruit

2 drops Rosemary

night-time arrival
2 drops Lavender

2 drops Geranium

2 drops Chamomile

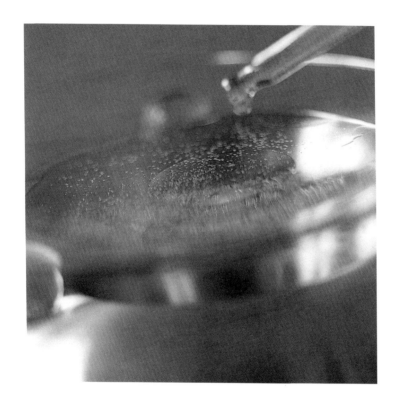

loss of smell

Essential oil of Basil is known to clear the sense of smell. If you feel you have become desensitised to smells, try using this recipe to recover.

6 drops Basil

memory loss

The healthier we are, the sharper our memory. Often, in times of transition, we recall lovely experiences from our past. Aromas help to evoke and revive memories, and good memories instil a sense of awareness of where you came from and where you are headed.

6 drops Rosemary

or

6 drops Peppermint

or

6 drops Basil

migraine

Many people suffer migraines caused by many different triggers. Marjoram oil is a traditional remedy for creating a more serene atmosphere in which to relax your mind and ground your body.

6 drops Marjoram

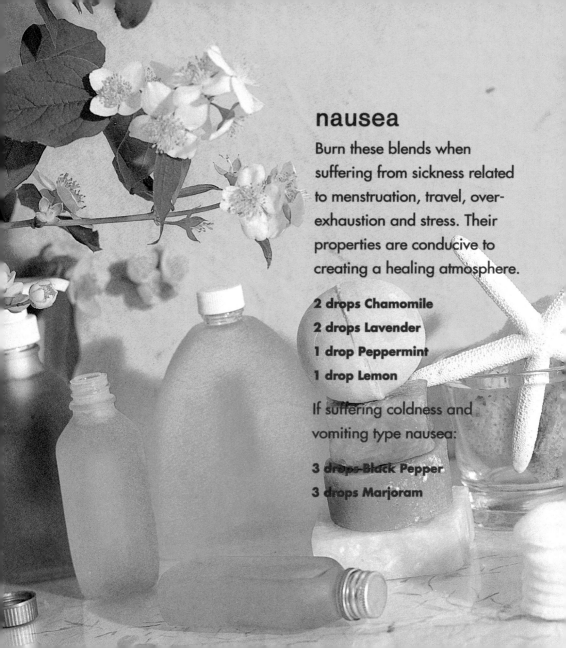

nausea

Burn these blends when suffering from sickness related to menstruation, travel, over-exhaustion and stress. Their properties are conducive to creating a healing atmosphere.

2 drops Chamomile
2 drops Lavender
1 drop Peppermint
1 drop Lemon

If suffering coldness and vomiting type nausea:

3 drops Black Pepper
3 drops Marjoram

opening chakras

Blends to burn to enliven the seven main energy centres of the body.
Chakras make up the core of our aura.

1 Crown Chakra. At the centre top of the head, this governs awareness, communication and spirituality.

2 Third-eye Chakra. In the middle of the forehead, this governs our inner intuition, logic and wisdom.

3 Throat Chakra. At the throat/neck area, this represents communication.

4 Heart Chakra. At the heart/lung area, this governs our destiny, love and emotions.

5 Solar Plexus Chakra. At the solar plexus/pancreas area, this rules our confidence, strength, perseverance, fear and joy.

6 Spleen Chakra. At the spleen and lower abdomen area, below the naval 'Hara', this controls digestion, stability, vitality and wisdom.

7 Base Chakra. At the reproductive area, this governs our sexuality, anger, spirituality and centredness.

2 drops Basil

2 drops Sage

2 drops Thyme

or

2 drops Nutmeg

2 drops Bay

2 drops Orange

pre-flight nerves

This blend of oils is highly recommended if you suffer from fear of flying. Light your aromatherapy burner and, breathing deeply and slowly, repeatedly visualise your plane taking off and landing safely. These oils will calm and centre you to help alleviate this fear.

4 drops Ginger

2 drops Peppermint

shock

When a traumatic event occurs in your life, the shock can affect your emotional and physical self. It may reveal itself in many ways including slight amnesia, hyperventilation, hysteria, severe depression and confusion. Aromatherapy is a wonderful way to calm yourself during the healing process of overcoming the immediate and long-term effects of shock. This blend is excellent for calming emotional grief and trauma. These oils carry uplifting properties that will help you to centre yourself and regain your strength. Rather than fight against your grief, allow your body to surrender and heal naturally.

3 drops Lavender

3 drops Peppermint

or

2 drops Peppermint

2 drops Melissa

2 drops Rosemary

strengthening

Being strong within makes you feel good, giving you the courage and persistence to overcome any hurdles in your way. This blend is beneficial for when you need to spend time alone to recover your inner spirit and focus on your positive attributes. These oils will help cleanse negative thoughts and comfort you in times of transition and change. Known to enhance energy and endurance, this is a good remedy to burn when you require that extra willpower to follow through.

2 drops Rosemary

2 drops Tea-tree

3 drops Cypress

toxic eliminators

Ridding the body of toxins is a challenging but immensely healing process. During the detoxification period, when you may experience fatigue and mood swings, burn these blends to create a positive and restful atmosphere for your healing.

3 drops Tea-tree

3 drops Lavender

or

3 drops Bergamot

3 drops Lemon

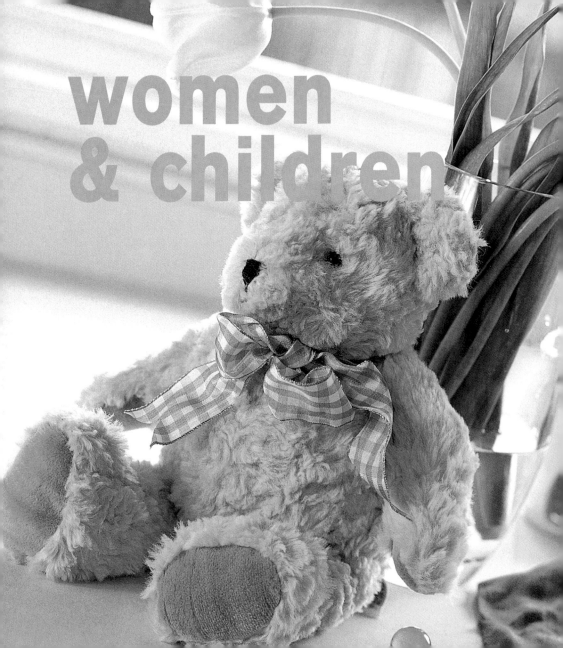

women
& children

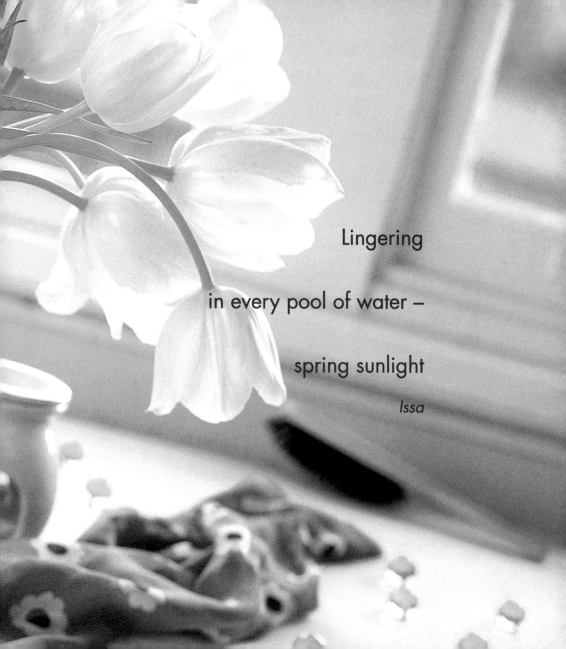

Lingering

in every pool of water –

spring sunlight

Issa

The time is ripe to celebrate the real beauty of women and their qualities of wisdom, intuition, understanding and the ability to speak and nurture from the heart. The blends in this section have been created to help deal with a range of women's special needs and to offer comfort during particular experiences.

sacred potion

These rich, intoxicating blends can be used to celebrate a very special experience or relationship. Carrying uplifting and aphrodisiac qualities, they work to honour spirituality, sensuality, devotion and love.

6 drops Rose Otto

or

4 drops pure Jasmine

2 drops Mandarin

premenstrual stress

If you suffer premenstrual stress, try to maximise your healthy lifestyle with good food and plenty of exercise. Burn these blends to help you relax. If you suffer severe repetitive premenstrual stress, seek advice from a reputable health practitioner.

3 drops Cypress
3 drops Juniper
or
3 drops Peppermint
3 drops Basil

For irritability and tearfulness:

3 drops Clary Sage
3 drops Marjoram

period pain (dysmenorrhoea)

Over fifty per cent of women suffer symptoms varying from slight discomfort to acute pain when they get their period. Usually the pain is in the first two days of the cycle. Take care to nurture yourself with warming baths and gentle massage. Do consult with a health practitioner if the pain you experience increases and occurs frequently.

2 drops Clary Sage
2 drops Fennel
1 drop Ylang Ylang
1 drop Neroli
or
3 drops Peppermint
3 drops Basil

menopause

Between the ages of 40–55, most women experience menopause, a time when menstrual bleeding comes to an end and the ovaries gradually decrease in function. Some women find this a liberating time, a phase of new experiences to accept and embrace with gratitude and grace. However, symptoms of this hormonal change can sometimes include hot flushes, mood swings, irritability and headaches. These blends will help to relax you during such times.

3 drops Geranium
3 drops Fennel

hot flushes

These lovely aromas will help to cool and calm your emotions after hot flushes. Known for their positive and comforting properties, they will encourage feelings of balance and openness to assist you during these experiences. Soaking your feet in a cool footbath is also a helpful way of reducing your temperature.

3 drops Clary Sage
3 drops Lime

morning sickness

Surrender to the journey of pregnancy and nurture yourself on all levels. These comforting oils can help to alleviate the nausea that can accompany pregnancy.

3 drops Lavender

3 drops Fennel

miscarriage

Whatever the reason for the loss of a child, healing yourself from the grief and hurt is a priority. These gentle aromas help to create a caring and compassionate environment. They encourage inner strength, harmony and peacefulness that can assist in the letting go process.

2 drops Lavender

2 drops Bergamot

2 drops Rose Otto

childbirth

Here are some oils to welcome and rejoice with a newborn child. These sensual oils also carry properties that are known to soothe panic and excitement. They are perfect to burn while you embrace this new being with love and joy.

6 drops Lavender

or

6 drops Jasmine

or any uplifting essential oil like Ylang Ylang, Rose or Neroli

post-natal blues

Many women experience some sort of low energy and emotion after the experience of giving birth. The following aromatic oils will help to soothe any low moments. Together they will relax the mind, rejuvenating feelings of self-confidence and happiness to give you the strength to take on your role as mother.

3 drops Neroli

2 drops Orange

1 drop Melissa

or

3 drops Grapefruit

3 drops Palma Rosa

Children are so spontaneous and playful that just spending time with them is healing. They need lots of love and nourishment and the freedom to develop and rely on their own inner voice. Use these blends to celebrate the time you spend with your own or others' children, whether at birthday parties or at bathtime and bedtime.

newborn's first days

This blend is perfect for both child and parents. Its balancing and calming properties fill the room with a lovely, relaxing aroma to induce peace and harmony.

2 drops Geranium
2 drops Lavender
2 drops Bergamot

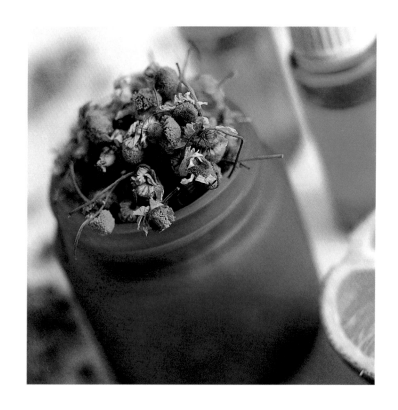

evening

Wonderful to burn for settling and reassuring children at night, these oils contain mild sedative qualities to encourage sleep. They will calm the emotions that cause restlessness in children, and are also ideal to burn for taming tantrums.

3 drops Sandalwood

3 drops Ylang Ylang

or

3 drops Chamomile

3 drops Bergamot

daytime

Burn this blend during the day to ignite a cheerful spark in children, and to encourage a peaceful yet inspiring atmosphere in which youngsters can happily play.

2 drops Lavender

2 drops Mandarin

2 drops Geranium

bathtime

These aromatic blends will help to create a joyful atmosphere while you and your children enjoy the bathing ritual.
Evening baths are a time when children can relax, connect with their family and talk about the events of the day. In the morning, these blends will add an invigorating spark to start the day.

3 drops Geranium
3 drops Bergamot
or
3 drops Palma Rosa
3 drops Cedarwood

storytime

Burn these blends to inspire your child's imagination. A mixture of soothing and refreshing aromas, they will awaken a child's senses, encouraging mental liveliness and joy. They also induce calmness so children can feel relaxed and enjoy their creative moments.

3 drops Orange
3 drops Sandalwood
or
3 drops Lavender
3 drops Geranium

bedtime

Specifically blended to seduce your child into a calming and restful sleep, Chamomile and Lavender are well-known for their sedating and comforting aromas.

3 drops Lavender

3 drops Chamomile

birthday party

These blends are great to calm and soothe the moods of over-excited kids. Burn this blend an hour before the party to fill the room with a happy atmosphere.

3 drops Geranium

3 drops Lavender

or

3 drops Bergamot

3 drops Petitgrain

school days

Children can become anxious as well as excited when they first start school, and can often find the long days tiring. Burn these blends before or after school to calm your child, yet encourage mental alertness and concentration.

3 drops Peppermint

3 drops Clary Sage

or

3 drops Rosemary

3 drops Lemon

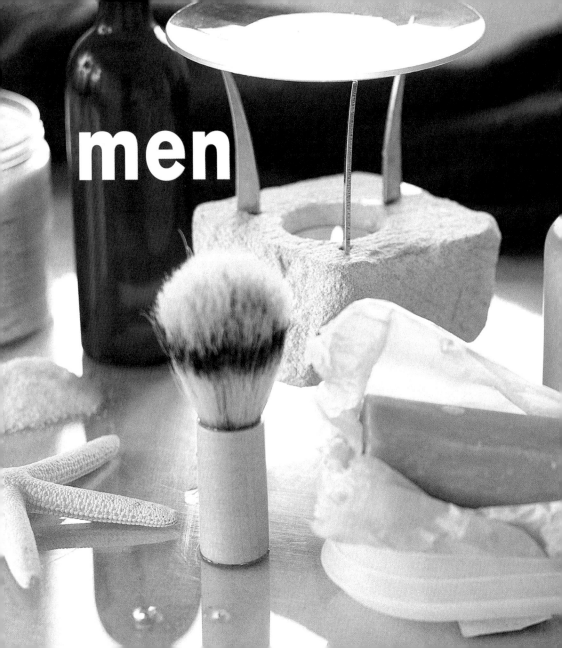

men

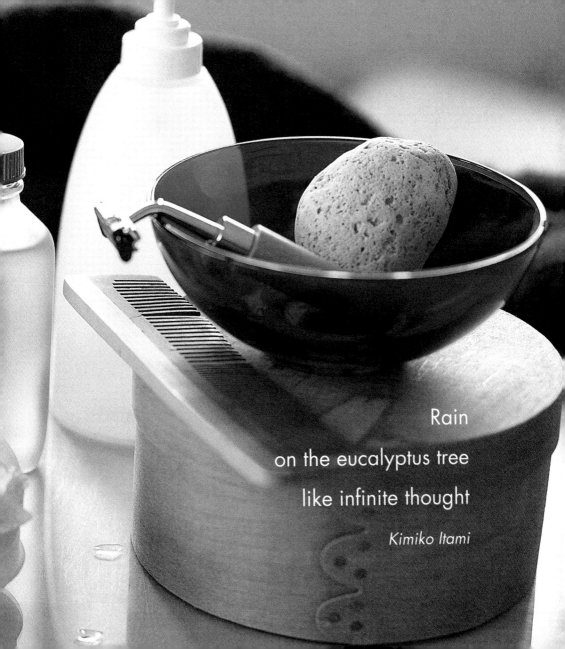

Rain
on the eucalyptus tree
like infinite thought

Kimiko Itami

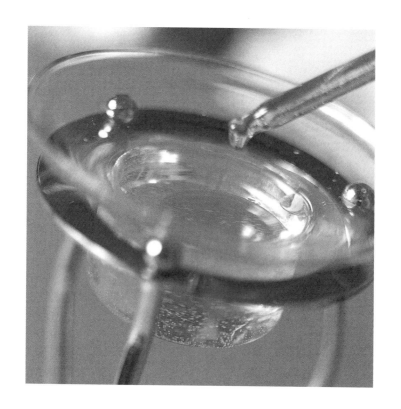

This section contains blends created especially for men and their personal needs. They celebrate men's unique qualities including their strength, depth, perception and intellect. Honouring the physical, spiritual and emotional beauty of men, these blends can help to both strengthen and soften emotions.

the warrior within

Awaken your inner wisdom, vision and spirit. These grounding blends will uplift and empower you as you grow in the process of awakening the warrior within. Known to nurture willpower and alleviate feelings of loss of self-esteem, they will bring you a positive and empowering energy, helping to build the confidence to break out and embrace your own energy.

warming
3 drops Clary Sage
3 drops Vetiver

cooling
3 drops Pine
3 drops Cypress

male energy

Enhance the characteristics of 'yang' energy for times when you need that extra stamina and courage to help you through the day. These positive oils will help inspire confidence and motivation, alleviating any 'stuck' feelings like frustration and resentment. Burn them when you feel mentally tired and need a boost of strong and powerfully centred energy.

3 drops Black Pepper
3 drops Grapefruit
or
3 drops Coriander
3 drops Ginger

stress relief

Take a break from your mind and let go of the feelings that you need to work, achieve and succeed in order to feel secure in life. To maintain your energy and health and really enjoy life, introduce some stress-relieving activities into your lifestyle. Spend some time walking, exercising or meditating. These blends are renowned for their lovely tranquil aromas, and will help with insomnia, fatigue and fear — all symptoms of stress.

2 drops Chamomile
2 drops Lavender
2 drops Petitgrain
or
2 drops Lemongrass
2 drops Mandarin
2 drops Neroli

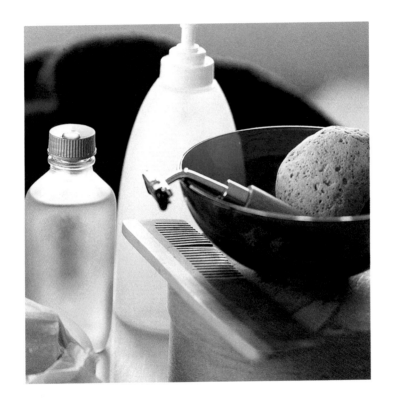

mental alertness

Burn these blends before an important meeting, an exam, or when you want to create an atmosphere where your friends and family can enjoy stimulating conversation. These oils can help to increase levels of focus and alertness, unblocking stagnant energy to make way for creative and imaginative thinking.

2 drops Frankincense
2 drops Cedarwood
2 drops Juniper
or
2 drops Coriander
2 drops Rosemary
2 drops Bergamot

sport and exercise

These vibrant and refreshing blends are for burning before or after sport and exercise. Their qualities will enhance energy and alertness, sharpening your responses and empowering you. They promote clear-thinking and assertiveness, but will also help to relax feelings of inadequacy and egoism, so games can be enjoyed that much more.

2 drops Cypress
2 drops Pine
2 drops Rosemary
or
2 drops Peppermint
2 drops Lavender
2 drops Eucalyptus

social occasions

These aromatic oils will promote positive, uplifting energy, and are especially great to burn at barbecues and outdoor gatherings. They are known to enhance feelings of security and confidence, to help generate relaxed and easy conversation. Refreshing and invigorating, they will also recharge and uplift everyone's mood, contributing to an enjoyable social occasion.

3 drops Rosewood
3 drops Geranium
or
3 drops Cinnamon
3 drops Clove

opening up

Communicating intimate feelings and thoughts can sometimes be difficult for many people. Being clear and honest about what you feel helps to affirm your self-worth and also allows you to feel comfortable with the intimacy required to build long-lasting friendships and relationships. Burn these refreshing blends when you feel you need a boost to bring your true thoughts and feelings to the surface.

3 drops Peppermint
3 drops Lemon
or
3 drops Juniper
3 drops Lime

father-to-be

Celebrate and enjoy this experience of intense excitement with these uplifting blends. Their beautiful scent will enhance this wonderful occasion of welcoming your child into the world, and help you to relax and give your partner your full support.

For the anxious father

3 drops Cedarwood

3 drops Bergamot

To cleanse the auric field before meeting your child

3 drops Lemon

3 drops Basil

male sexuality

Qualities of male sexuality include protectiveness, endurance, vigour and comfort. All men can be beautiful lovers — playful and seductive with a genuine deep warmth and love. These blends are to invigorate and stimulate the mood, strengthening a man's sexuality.

3 drops Frankincense

3 drops Myrrh

or

3 drops Palma Rosa

3 drops Cinnamon

masculine aphrodisiac

Create an aura of desire and sensuality around yourself. Whether it be flirtatious and fun or self-assured and earthy, these aromas will help stimulate all the senses. Calming and harmonious, the oils will also give rise to a mood that honours the compassionate side of male sexuality.

2 drops Vetiver
2 drops Rosewood
2 drops Patchouli

impotence

Burning these soothing blends, getting a massage and taking a bath will help to centre and relax you to enjoy lovemaking. Connect with your partner on a deeper level through open and honest communication and you may find your heart softening to embrace this sensual experience.

3 drops Juniper
2 drops Lavender
1 drop Sandalwood
or
3 drops Rose Otto
3 drops Lavender

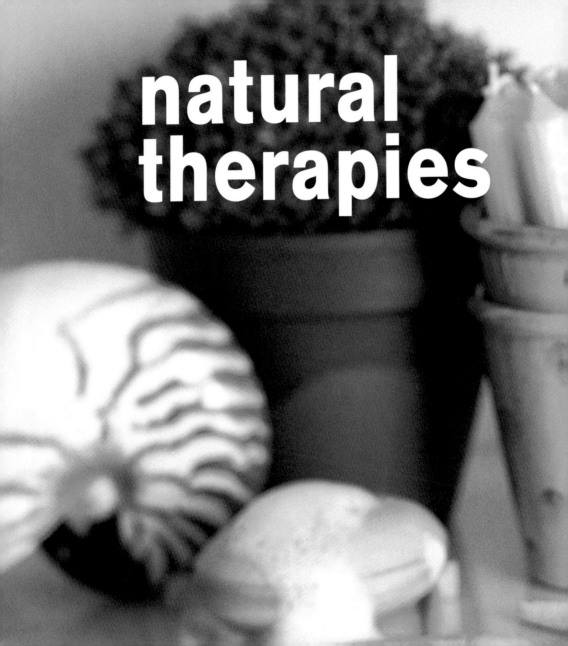

natural
therapies

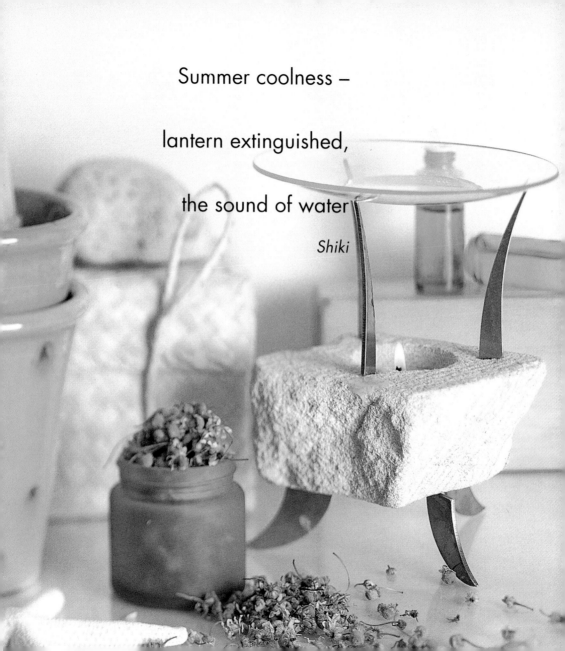

Summer coolness –

lantern extinguished,

the sound of water

Shiki

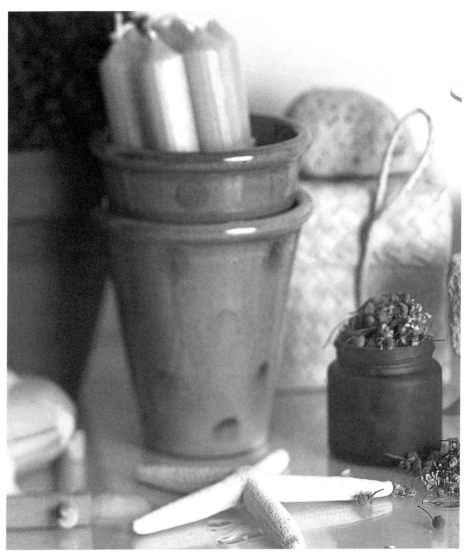

'Natural therapies' are natural ways of caring for and healing the causes of physical and emotional problems. They include aromatherapy, massage, reflexology, traditional Chinese medicine, homeopathy, nutrition and naturopathy.

Through the study of natural therapies, we can learn how to manage our own physical, emotional and mental health. For example, we will be able to recognise signs of ill-health before we get sick. If a friend has a headache, we can offer to massage them to relieve the pain. If we suffer from sleeplessness, maybe a simple yoga posture will help us relax. Ultimately, we can understand that recovery from illness starts within.

The blends in this section are created to burn when studying, practising or receiving some sort of natural healing.

massage

Massage therapy can be looked upon not only as a luxury, but as an essential part of a health regime. Regular massage is a great reliever of many ills. It can free unresolved traumas stored in the body and help us to relieve tension. It is a wonderful way to relax completely to help the healing process take place.

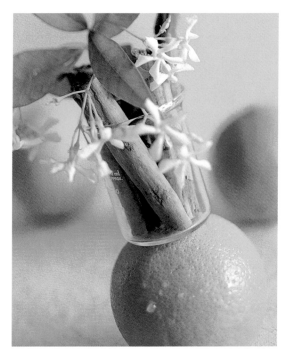

Here are some special blends to accompany
your favourite style of massage:

shiatsu

An invigorating combination
of oils to move energy and
stimulate circulation.

3 drops Ginger

3 drops Marjoram

swedish

Oils known to revitalise and
strengthen your energy.

2 drops Rosemary

2 drops Basil

2 drops Peppermint

sensual

The perfect blend to intensify
feelings of intimacy and
physical closeness.

2 drops Clary Sage

2 drops Patchouli

2 drops Orange

stress-release

A relaxing mix to relieve
tensions and impart a sense
of youth and vitality.

2 drops Lavender

2 drops Chamomile

2 drops Sandalwood

yoga

Many people say yoga saved their lives by helping them when they felt stuck and static, bringing new meaning and fresh purpose to their lives. Yoga works like an inner shower, cleansing and energising vital organs and bodily functions. Regular yoga practice is one of the most effective methods known for ongoing health maintenance.

Here are two proven blends to support your yoga routines.

morning yoga
2 drops Lemongrass

2 drops Orange

2 drops Bergamot

evening yoga
2 drops Rosemary

2 drops Thyme

2 drops Lavender

meditation

The practice of meditation can bring you the incomparable experience of pure stillness, putting you in touch with your true essence and your potential as a human being. Frankincense and Myrrh have traditionally been used to support meditation — but remember not to make the aroma so overpowering that it interferes with the meditative process.

3 drops Frankincense

3 drops Myrrh

or

6 drops Frankincense only

or

6 drops Myrrh only

or

6 drops Cypress only

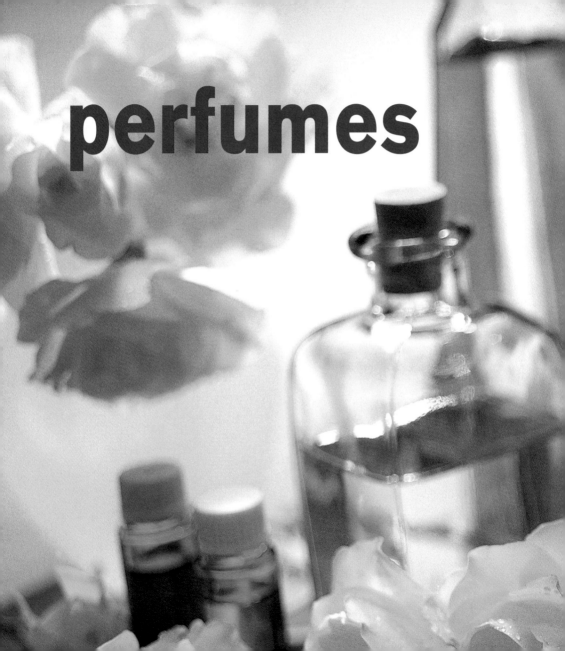

perfumes

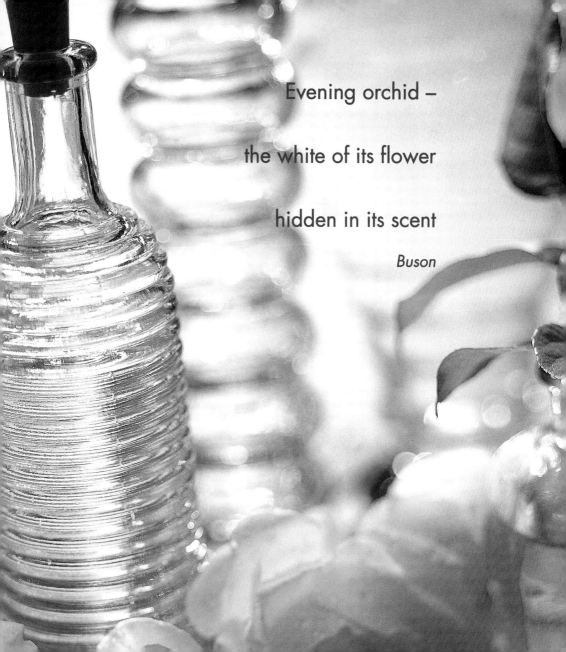

Evening orchid –

the white of its flower

hidden in its scent

Buson

Create your own pure perfumes without the chemicals used in many commercial perfumes today. These blends will circulate special aromas in the home, lifting the spirits of anyone who enters. Be creative with these oils and use your intuition to make up your own perfumes by choosing aromas you enjoy.

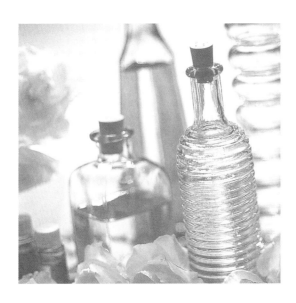

floral

3 drops Ylang Ylang

2 drops Geranium

1 drop Neroli

or

3 drops Cedarwood

2 drops Lavender

1 drop Mandarin

spicy

3 drops Peppermint

3 drops Clove

or

3 drops Rosemary

3 drops Coriander

woody

3 drops Vetiver

3 drops Cedarwood

or

3 drops Clary Sage

3 drops Sandalwood

sweet

4 drops Ylang Ylang

2 drops Grapefruit

or

3 drops Neroli

3 drops Geranium

masculine (yang)

3 drops Cinnamon

3 drops Aniseed

or

3 drops Sandalwood

3 drops Lemon

ocean

2 drops Geranium

2 drops Ylang Ylang

2 drops Cedarwood

in Rosewater base

feminine (yin)

3 drops Bergamot

3 drops Vanilla

or

1 drop Rose Otto

2 drops Geranium

3 drops Melissa

forest

2 drops Pine

2 drops Hyssop

2 drops Eucalyptus

1 drop Cypress

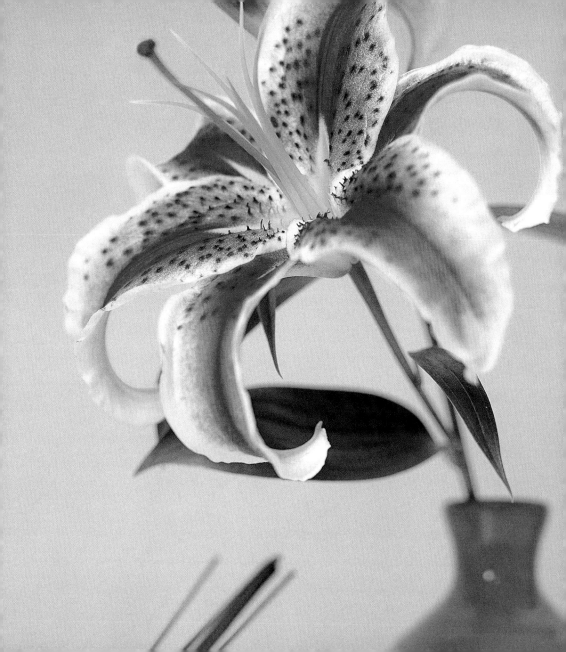

cool down

Vaporise these blends when summer's heat is extreme and you need to bring a cooler quality into your home or workplace. These blends will help create an atmosphere that is light, refreshing and energised.

3 drops Peppermint

3 drops Lime

or

3 drops Lavender

3 drops Geranium

warm up

For burning when you and your home feel chilled, these blends will create the impression of a warmer temperature, igniting a glow and circulating the subtle essences of calmness and joy.

3 drops Mandarin

3 drops Black Pepper

or

3 drops Cinnamon

3 drops Orange

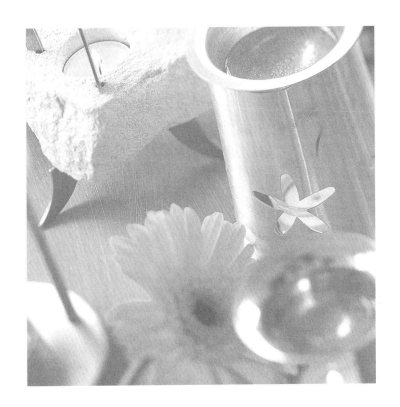

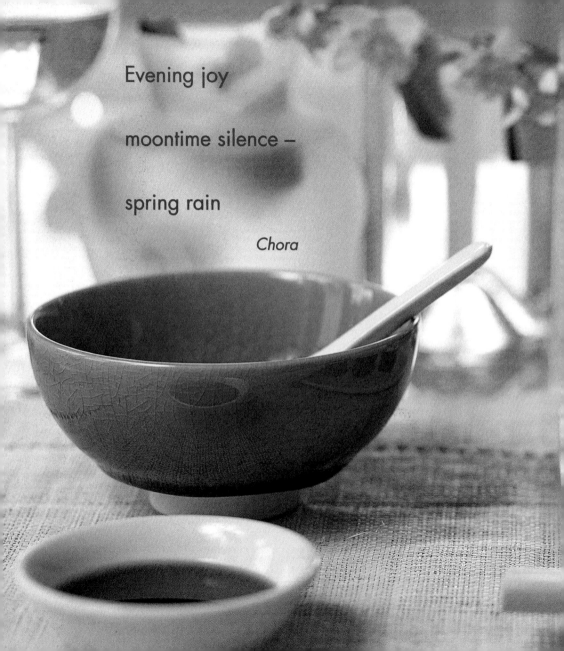

Evening joy

moontime silence –

spring rain

Chora

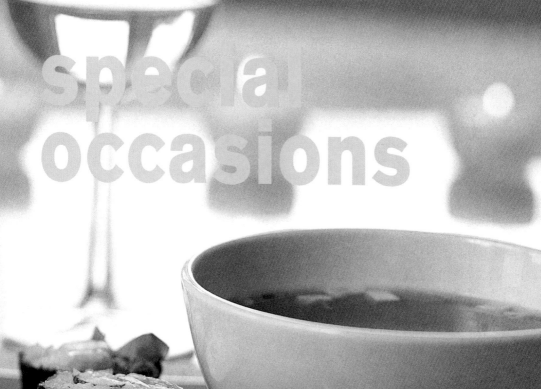

special
occasions

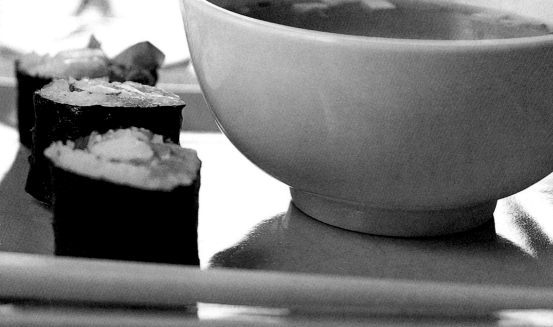

The new seasons and other special occasions bring new experiences, interests, places and people to meet. Celebrating their arrival with parties and gatherings is a lovely way to lift the spirits of friends and family. Aromatherapy is a magical way to honour the love and friendship between people as well as simply celebrate the beauty and nature of life itself.

spring

Celebrate romance, beauty, hope, love, idealism, vitality, exoticism, spirit, enthusiasm, colour and growth.

3 drops Melissa

3 drops Grapefruit

or

3 drops Mandarin

3 drops Black Pepper

summer

Celebrate sensuality, sun, sand, water, playfulness, rejuvenation, liberty, leisure, lucidity, freshness, vigour and sex.

3 drops Lemon

3 drops Bergamot

or

3 drops Pine

3 drops Cypress

autumn

Celebrate depth, warmth, reflection, seduction, lavishness, synergy, temptation, belief, hope, stillness and resurrection.

3 drops Cedarwood

3 drops Petitgrain

or

3 drops Sandalwood

3 drops Lavender

winter

Celebrate falling leaves, fire and ice, mental activity, creativity, loyalty, memory, strength, potency and festivity.

3 drops Clove

3 drops Ginger

or

3 drops Cinnamon

3 drops Orange

spring equinox

The time of year when winter moves to spring. A time for celebrations of all kinds including traditional planting festivals.

3 drops Patchouli

3 drops Vetiver

or

4 drops Mandarin

2 drops Frankincense

autumn equinox

Traditionally the time of harvesting the crops. These blends celebrate the moving of summer into autumn.

3 drops Cedarwood

3 drops Pine

or

3 drops Clary Sage

3 drops Juniper

full moon

At the full moon, moods intensify, dramatic events occur and you may find you have difficulty sleeping. These blends will induce calmness at such times.

3 drops Clary Sage
3 drops Ylang Ylang
or
3 drops Geranium
3 drops Lavender

christmas

Enhance the spirit of Christmas with a mixture of essential oils to fill the room with aromas of wood, spice, warmth and good cheer.

2 drops Frankincense
2 drops Myrrh
2 drops Sandalwood
or
2 drops Cinnamon
2 drops Orange
2 drops Clove

wedding

These sacred blends of very special oils celebrate the connection of two people taking the step to commit their love and truth to each other.

2 drops Geranium

2 drops Ylang Ylang

2 drops Vanilla

or

3 drops Jasmine

3 drops Ginger

st. valentine's day

Celebrate love and romance on this traditional day for lovers of all ages.

3 drops Carnation Absolute

3 drops Cedarwood

or

2 drops Petitgrain

2 drops Ylang Ylang

2 drops Sandalwood

or

3 drops Patchouli

3 drops Geranium

parties

spring/summer

An exquisite refreshing and uplifting aroma to welcome with open arms the warmth of spring and summer — the seasons of sand, surf, sun and tropical fruits.

3 drops Lime

3 drops Lemongrass

autumn/winter

Bring back the warm memories of bright leaves, crisp air and snow. This delicious sweet aroma welcomes the cold with a smile.

3 drops Vanilla

3 drops Cinnamon

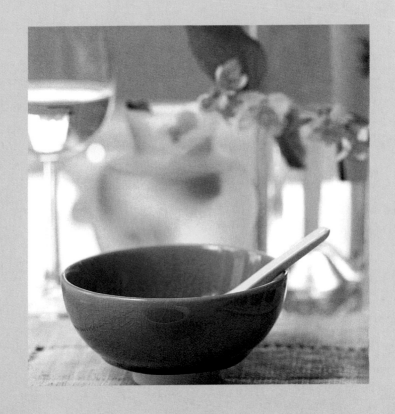

dinner parties

Match essential oils to the food you are cooking so when
your guests enter the room they are instantly immersed
in the atmosphere of the evening's cuisine.

asian

3 drops Aniseed

3 drops Grapefruit

australian

2 drops Lemon Myrtle

2 drops Eucalyptus

1 drop Tea-tree

japanese

3 drops Orange

2 drops Lemon

1 drop Eucalyptus

1 drop Cinnamon

thai

3 drops Lemongrass

3 drops Lime

indian

2 drops Ginger

2 drops Cinnamon

2 drops Clove

or

2 drops Sandalwood

2 drops Clove

2 drops Cinnamon

european

2 drops Orange

2 drops Neroli

1 drop Ylang Ylang

1 drop Geranium

vegetarian

6 drops Sandalwood

vegan

3 drops Fennel

3 drops Marjoram

3 drops Thyme

3 drops Lemon

mexican

3 drops Ginger

3 drops Lemon

macrobiotic

3 drops Cypress

3 drops Vetiver

or

3 drops Thyme

3 drops Lemon

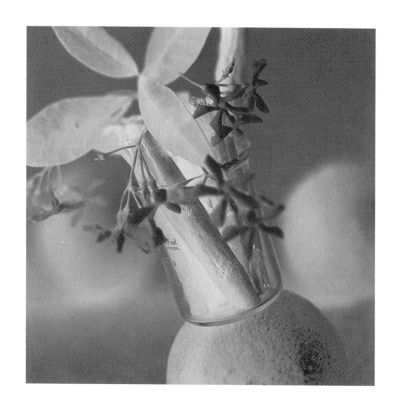

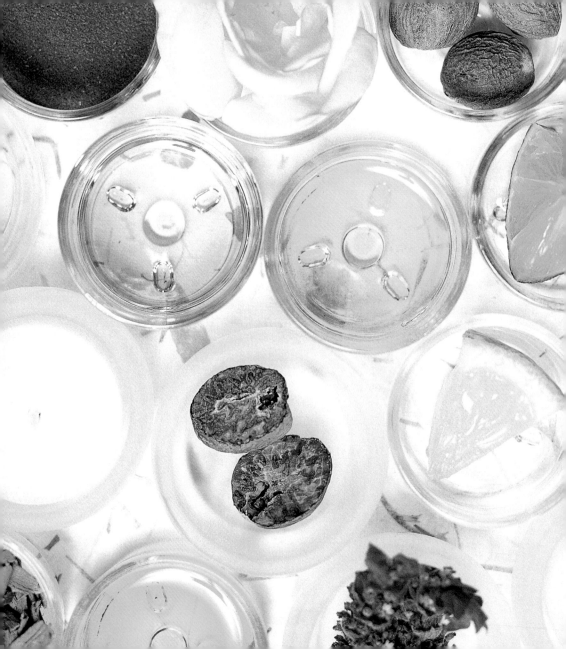

glossary of oils

Essential oils have many properties and can be used in many different ways: in massage, baths, compresses, ointments and mouthwashes.
The blends in this book are for vaporisation only.
  Be creative and have fun with your oils, and experiment with creating your own blends.
If you find you don't like an oil, don't use it.

angelica

Angelica archangelica

AVOID DURING PREGNANCY

Method of extraction	Steam distillation of the seeds
Enhances	Higher energy, inspiration, emotional strength, encouragement, support, alertness
Reduces	Fatigue, stress, respiratory problems, migraine, impatience, apathy, feelings of weakness, timidity

aniseed

Pimpinella anisum

Method of extraction	Steam distillation of the seeds
Enhances	Higher energy and rejuvenation
Reduces	Respiratory problems, mental fatigue

basil

Ocimum basilicum

AVOID DURING PREGNANCY

Method of extraction	Steam distillation of the leaves and flowers
Enhances	Assertiveness, concentration, trust, happiness, purpose, balance, clarity of thought, decision-making, relaxation
Reduces	Depression, anxiety, mental fatigue, respiratory problems, scanty menstruation, loss of smell, insomnia, nervous tension, fever, nausea, hysteria, indecision

bay
Pimenta racemosa

Method of extraction	Steam distillation of the leaves
Enhances	Energy, expression, confidence, creativity, courage, the heart, sensuality
Reduces	Bronchial colds and flu, poor communication

benzoin
Styrax benzoin

USE ONLY IN SMALL AMOUNTS

Method of extraction	Resin from the bark
Enhances	Energy, calmness, confidence, protectiveness, consciousness, warmth, cleansing of air, self-empowerment, healing, openness, deep sleep, deep breathing, relaxation
Reduces	Stress, emotional exhaustion, indifference, anxiety, depression, anger, loneliness, shyness, crisis, sadness, past resentments and tensions, stagnation, respiratory problems

bergamot
Citrus bergamia

Method of extraction	Cold expression from the rind of the bergamot orange
Enhances	Positive energy, calmness, relaxation, concentration, confidence, letting go, balance, motivation, completion, joy, rejuvenation, strength, fulfilment
Reduces	Depression, anxiety, listlessness, weakened spirit, burn-out, stress, loneliness, grief, tension, bitterness, sadness

black pepper

Piper nigrum

Method of extraction	Steam distillation of the dried fruits (peppercorns)
Enhances	Clarity of thought, endurance, security, comfort, motivation, communication, direction, decision-making, aphrodisiac, confronting your fears
Reduces	Emotional blocks, anger, indecision, mental fatigue, nervousness, indifference, frustration, vagueness, stress

cajuput

Melaleuca cajuputi

Method of extraction	Steam distillation of the leaves, buds and twigs
Enhances	Higher energy, mental stimulation, centredness, wellbeing, clarity of thought
Reduces	Respiratory problems, mental fatigue, apathy, cynicism, procrastination

calendula

Calendula officinalis

Method of extraction	Infused
Enhances	Calmness, relaxation
Reduces	Inner loneliness, emotional wounds, good for children

cardamon

Elettaria cardamomum

Method of extraction	Steam distillation of the seeds
Enhances	Clarity of thought, fulfilment, concentration, confidence, motivation, sensuality, joy, caring, courage, willpower, inspiration, warming
Reduces	Stress, mental fatigue, nervous exhaustion, thoughtlessness, uneasiness, restricted thoughts, judgemental feelings, distrust, fear

carnation absolute

Dianthus caryophyllus

Method of extraction	Solvent extraction of the flowers
Enhances	Expression, warmth, self-esteem, imagination, trust, honesty, aphrodisiac
Reduces	Negativity, loneliness, suspicion, fear, worry, listlessness

cedarwood

Juniperus virginiana

AVOID DURING PREGNANCY

Method of extraction	Steam distillation of the wood chips and leaves
Enhances	Calmness, emotional release, positiveness, balance, sexuality, harmony, confidence, focus, security, self-empowerment, mental relaxation, emotional strength, caring, endurance
Reduces	Negativity, depression, insomnia, fear, respiratory problems, premenstrual stress, tension, vagueness, excitability, aggression, over-sensitivity, distrust, obsession, conflict

chamomile

Matricaria chamomilla (German)
Anthemis nobilis (Roman)

AVOID DURING FIRST THREE MONTHS OF PREGNANCY

Chamomile oil is very expensive, so it is more economical to buy it diluted in a carrier oil.

Method of extraction	Steam distillation of the flowers
Enhances	Healing, peace, positiveness, understanding, releasing past emotions, relaxation, stability, communication, balanced emotions, spirituality
Reduces	Stress, depression, impatience, nerves, insomnia, hysteria, over-sensitivity, resentment

cinnamon

Cinnamomum zeylanicum

Method of extraction	Steam distillation of the leaves
Enhances	Healing, spirituality, sensuality, awareness, security, stability, concentration, rejuvenation, warming
Reduces	Depression, mental fatigue, tension, fear, sensitivity to the hardness of life, resentment, shallowness, hatred

citronella

Cymbopogon nardus

Citronella makes an excellent insect repellent.

Method of extraction	Steam distillation of the dried leaves
Enhances	Creativity, emotional strength, clarity of thought, inspiration
Reduces	Depression, lack of motivation, cluttered mind

clary sage

Salvia sclarea

AVOID DURING PREGNANCY

Method of extraction	Steam distillation of the leaves
Enhances	Calmness, sexuality, wellbeing, relaxation, expansion, clarity of thought, creativity, inspiration, tranquillity, balance, vitality, confidence, euphoria, communication
Reduces	Respiratory problems, irregular menstruation, nervous tension, stress, depression, migraine, over-excitement, suspicion, vagueness, fear, mental fatigue, guilt, obsessiveness, tearfulness, frigidity

clove

Eugenia caryophyllata

Method of extraction	Steam distillation of the leaves
Enhances	Mental alertness, balanced emotions, memory, endurance, security, calmness, decision-making, assertiveness, sensuality
Reduces	Mental fatigue, loss of direction, emotional weakness, feelings of failure, loss of confidence

coriander

Coriandrum sativum

Method of extraction	Steam distillation of the seeds
Enhances	Motivation, confidence, memory, communication, positive energy, creative inspiration, vitality, excitement, honesty
Reduces	Colds and flu, mental fatigue, forgetfulness, stress, nervous tension, self-doubt, frustration

cypress

Cupressus sempervirens

Method of extraction	Steam distillation of the leaves, cones and twigs
Enhances	Calmness, letting go, accepting change, strength, assertiveness, honesty, solitude, self-empowerment, inner wisdom, decisiveness, harmony
Reduces	Respiratory problems, menopausal problems, nervous tension, stress, excessive menstruation, grief, impatience, sadness, loss of direction, distrust, fear, imbalance, resentment, loneliness

eucalyptus

Eucalyptus globulus

Method of extraction	Steam distillation of the leaves
Enhances	Healing, protectiveness, concentration, vitality, balanced emotions, mental clarity, spontaneity
Reduces	Respiratory problems, fevers, headache, mental clarity, confrontations, irrational behaviour, anger, insect repellent, bad odours

fennel

Foeniculum vulgare

Method of extraction	Steam distillation of the seeds
Enhances	Happiness, perseverance, confidence, emotional release, relaxation, creativity, courage, security, rejuvenation, spirituality, assertiveness, ambition
Reduces	Loss of menstruation, nausea, menopausal problems, conflict, rigidity, fear, lack of energy and interest for life, stagnation

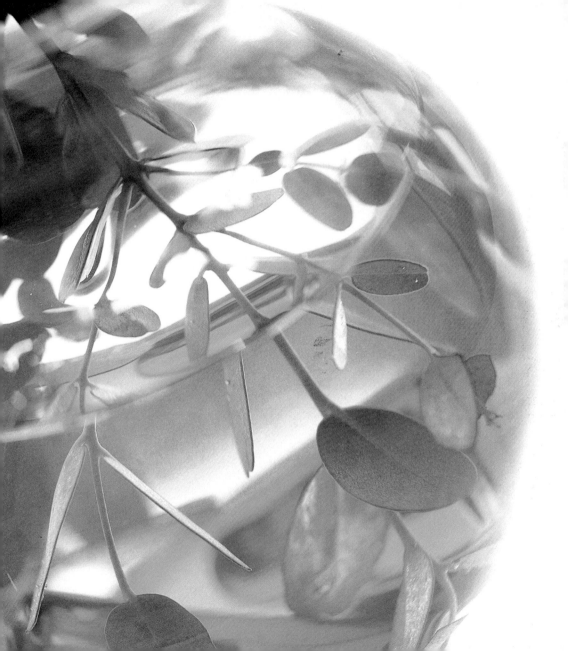

frankincense
Boswellia thurifera
AVOID DURING FIRST THREE MONTHS OF PREGNANCY

Method of extraction	Steam distillation of the gum-resin
Enhances	Calmness, spirituality, balance, meditation, warming, healing, security, inner wisdom, courage,emotional release
Reduces	Respiratory problems, painful menstruation, stress, insomnia, emotional weakness, fear, exhaustion, imbalance, sorrow, dishonesty, obsession

geranium
Pelargonium graveolens

Method of extraction	Steam distillation of the leaves
Enhances	Calmness, balance, comfort, laughter, social occasions, security, self-confidence, decisiveness, logical thought, contentment, ability to change
Reduces	Menopausal problems, stress, premenstrual stress, depression, insect repellent, anxiety, lack of self-control, rigidity, mood swings, traumatic experiences both past and present, stagnation

ginger
Zingiber officinale

Method of extraction	Steam distillation of the roots
Enhances	Decisiveness, courage, confidence, strength, mental clarity, memory, sexuality, vitality, understanding, warmth, endurance
Reduces	Coughs, nausea, travel sickness, colds and flu, mental fatigue, impotence, loneliness, confusion, sadness, loss of direction, apathy

grapefruit
Citrus paradisi

Method of extraction	Steam distillation of the peel
Enhances	Balance, positive energy, confidence, joy, vitality, spontaneity, courage, security, clarity of thought, self-empowerment, inspiration, creativity, cooperation
Reduces	Depression, colds and flu, exhaustion, indecisiveness, frustration, bitterness, insecurity, sadness, irritability

hyssop
Hyssopus officinalis

Method of extraction	Steam distillation of the leaves
Enhances	Relaxation, alertness, emotional sensibility, focus
Reduces	Sluggish mind, scattered thoughts, tension, sleeplessness

jasmine
Jasminum grandiflorum

AVOID DURING PREGNANCY

Pure Jasmine oil is very expensive, so buy Jasmine oil that is diluted in a carrier oil.

Method of extraction	Solvent extraction of the flowers
Enhances	Harmony, positiveness, sexuality, self-worth, sensitivity, inspiration, clarity of thought, hope, magic, assertiveness, openness, inner wisdom, calmness, joy, warmth, romance, love
Reduces	Depression, post-natal depression, anxiety, coughs, painful menstruation, stress, premenstrual stress, apathy, lack of confidence, moodiness, bitterness, envy, emotional stagnation, frigidity

juniper

Juniperus communis

AVOID DURING PREGNANCY

Method of extraction	Steam distillation of the ripe berries
Enhances	Positiveness, healing, calmness, centredness, inner wisdom, self-confidence, fulfilment, concentration, creativity, openness, meditation, warmth
Reduces	Loss of menstruation, premenstrual stress, nervous tension, sleeplessness, anxiety, insecurity, lack of vitality

lavender

Lavandula officinalis

Method of extraction	Steam distillation of the flowers
Enhances	Calmness, balance, healing, comfort, openness, acceptance, relaxation, spirituality, resolving of conflict, strengthening, decision-making
Reduces	Depression, stress, painful menstruation, insomnia, nervous tension, migraine, premenstrual stress, emotional imbalance, fear, hysteria, frustration, shock, panic, over-sensitivity, insect repellent

lemon

Citrus limon

Method of extraction	Cold expression from the peel
Enhances	Calmness, alertness, happiness, vitality, positiveness, laughter, motivation, decision-making, awareness, stability, ambition
Reduces	Respiratory problems, high blood pressure, forgetfulness, stress, lack of focus, apprehension, negative thoughts, bitterness, apathy, fear, mental strain, aloofness

lemon myrtle

Myrtus communis

Method of extraction	Steam distillation of the leaves
Enhances	Compassion, endurance, openness, willpower, vigour
Reduces	Intolerance, over-indulgence, lack of energy

lemon verbena

Lippia citriodora

Method of extraction	Steam distillation of the flower stalks
Enhances	Concentration, motivation, joy, recovery from illness
Reduces	Apathy, stagnation, low self-esteem, unhappiness

lemongrass

Cymbopogon citratus

Method of extraction	Steam distillation of the leaves
Enhances	Concentration, vitality, awareness, clarity of thought, rejuvenation
Reduces	Depression, mental exhaustion, stress, nervousness, over-active mind

lime

Citrus aurantifolia

Method of extraction	Cold expression from the peel
Enhances	Vitality, positive energy, clarity of thought, assertiveness, decisiveness, fun, laughter, appetite for life, inspiration
Reduces	Colds and flu, depression, nervous exhaustion, stress, fatigue, self-doubt, heaviness, apathy

mandarin

Citrus nobilis

Method of extraction	Cold expression from the peel
Enhances	Inspiration, gentleness, peacefulness, empathy, emotional strength, serenity, fulfilment, motivation, encouragement
Reduces	Insomnia, nervous tension, stress, panic, past traumas, anxiety, depression, sadness, excitability, restlessness

marjoram

Origanum marjorana

AVOID DURING PREGNANCY

Method of extraction	Steam distillation of the leaves
Enhances	Restful sleep, calmness, balance, courage, determination, comfort, self-confidence, focus, warmth
Reduces	Insomnia, nervous tension, premenstrual stress, painful menstruation, colds and flu, grief, agitation, loneliness, panic, anger, resentment

melissa

Melissa officinalis

Method of extraction	Steam distillation of the leaves
Enhances	Calmness, sensitivity, happiness, harmony, positiveness, vitality, enthusiasm, alertness, security, relaxation, self-acknowledgement, confidence, hope
Reduces	Depression, feelings of emptiness, anxiety, nervous exhaustion, insomnia, respiratory problems, grief, anger, excitability

myrrh

Commiphora myrrha

AVOID DURING PREGNANCY

Method of extraction	Steam distillation of the gum-resin
Enhances	Spirituality, inspiration, positiveness, magic, calmness, self-assurance, letting go, rejuvenation, faith
Reduces	Respiratory problems, over-sensitivity, despair, depression, uncertainty, anger

neroli

Citrus aurantium

Method of extraction	Steam distillation of the bitter orange flowers
Enhances	Centredness, self-confidence, sensuality, positive energy, fulfilment, love, empathy, peacefulness, happiness, relaxation
Reduces	Depression, anxiety, premenstrual stress, fear, shock, panic, sorrow, past traumas, feelings of emptiness

nutmeg

Myristica fragrans

AVOID DURING PREGNANCY

Method of extraction	Steam distillation of the dried kernel (nut)
Enhances	Enthusiasm, inspiration, playfulness, positive energy, vitality, mental stimulation, eroticism, seduction
Reduces	Nervousness, sexual fears, anxiety, mental exhaustion, self-doubt

orange

Citrus aurantium

Method of extraction	Cold expression from the peel
Enhances	Sexuality, sensuality, joy, creativity, balance, self-assurance, warmth, love, communication, vitality, positive energy, balance, courage, inspiration, encouragement, consideration, pleasure
Reduces	Depression, stress, anxiety, respiratory problems, insomnia, obsession, insecurity, sadness, past traumas, emotional wounds, mental exhaustion, apathy, loss of hope

palma rosa
Cymbopogon martinii

Method of extraction	Steam distillation of the dried leaves
Enhances	Clarity of thought, focus, love, vitality, balance, emotional strength
Reduces	Depression, nervous exhaustion, stress, anguish, apathy, restlessness

patchouli
Pogostemon patchouli

Method of extraction	Fermentation, then steam distillation of the dried leaves
Enhances	Positiveness, endurance, self-assurance, vitality, balance, consideration, gentleness, sexuality, fulfilment, purpose, laughter, wisdom, seduction, alertness, love, peacefulness
Reduces	Nervous exhaustion, stress, depression, sexual fears, insomnia, listlessness, over-sensitivity, anxiety, conflict, insect repellent

pennyroyal
Mentha pulegium

AVOID DURING PREGNANCY

Method of extraction	Steam distillation of the leaves
Enhances	Purification, positiveness, mental strength, openness, clearing
Reduces	Exhaustion, nervousness, hysteria, resentment

peppermint

Mentha piperita

AVOID DURING PREGNANCY

Method of extraction	Steam distillation of the leaves
Enhances	Concentration, vitality, self-confidence, emotional release, positiveness, sensuality, direction, clear thinking, self-empowerment
Reduces	Nausea, burn-out, shock, apathy, hysteria, colds and flu, headaches, lethargy, self-doubt, fear, vulnerabilty, insect repellent

petitgrain

Citrus aurantium

Method of extraction	Steam distillation of the leaves and twigs
Enhances	Hope, calmness, harmony, communication, self-assurance, emotional strength, friendship, security, balance, inspiration, wisdom, alertness, rejuvenation, openness
Reduces	Nervous exhaustion, stress, premenstrual stress, insomnia, anxiety, vulnerability, anger, insecurity, confusion, frustration, loss of hope, sadness, stagnation

pine

Pinus sylvestris

Method of extraction	Steam distillation of pine needles and twigs
Enhances	Self-empowerment, positive energy, wisdom, trust, honesty, love, joy, focus, security, inspiration, concentration, inner strength, empathy, letting go

Reduces	Self-doubt, stress, fatigue, colds and flu, respiratory problems, frigidity, apathy, impatience, anxiety, resentment, mental fatigue, depression, guilt, sorrow, boredom, confusion

rose

Rosa centifolia

Pure Rose oil is very expensive and is best purchased diluted in a carrier oil.

Method of extraction	Solvent extraction from the rose petals
Enhances	Healing, sensuality, femininity, understanding, love, peace, passion, warmth, confidence, happiness, security, motivation, rejuvenation, openness, fulfilment, compassion
Reduces	Depression, stress, insomnia, loss of confidence, grief, apathy, insecurity, vulnerability, sexual fears, envy, feelings of emptiness, anger

rose otto

Rosa damascena

Method of extraction	Steam distillation from the damask rose
Enhances	Love, harmony, happiness, comfort, tenderness, gratitude, wisdom, spiritual awareness, confidence, sensuality, enchantment
Reduces	Despair, anxiety, sorrow, vulnerability, guilt, shyness, over-sensitivity, emotional trauma, envy, broken heart, self-doubt

rosemary

Rosmarinus officinalis

AVOID DURING PREGNANCY

Method of extraction	Steam distillation of the leaves
Enhances	Concentration, clarity of thought, warmth, emotional strength, creative inspiration, self-empowerment, centring, stability, awareness, sensuality, confidence, honesty, positive energy, decisiveness, openness, remembrance
Reduces	Mental fatigue, depression, nervous exhaustion, stress, painful menstruation, colds and flu, respiratory problems, forgetfulness, confusion, indecision, insincerity, insect repellent

rosewood

Aniba rosaeodora

Method of extraction	Steam distillation of the heartwood
Enhances	Relaxation, vitality, positive energy, spirituality, security, serenity, focus, balance, sexual energy
Reduces	Nervousness, lack of concentration, mood swings, confusion, depression

sage

Salvia officinalis

AVOID DURING PREGNANCY

Method of extraction	Steam distillation of the leaves and flowers
Enhances	Healing, calmness, positiveness, balance, alertness, rejuvenation
Reduces	Depression, feelings of emptiness, anxiety, forgetfulness, fatigue, sorrow, bad odours

sandalwood

Santalum album

Method of extraction | Steam distillation of the heartwood

Enhances | Centring, openness, meditation, warmth, self-assurance, honesty, tranquillity, love, spirituality, sensuality, healing, comfort, hope, faith, inner wisdom, understanding, togetherness, stability, courage, endurance

Reduces | Depression, premenstrual stress, insomnia, stress, sleeplessness, impotence, lack of concentration, despair, obsession, irritability, self-doubt, apprehension, scepticism, loneliness, past traumas

spearmint

Mentha spicata

Method of extraction | Steam distillation of the leaves

Enhances | Calmness, clarity, focus, compassion

Reduces | Respiratory problems, resentment, selfishness

tea-tree

Melaleuca alternifolia

Method of extraction | Steam distillation of the leaves

Enhances | Courage, confidence, mental clarity, cleansing, energising

Reduces | Colds and flu, respiratory problems, lack of confidence, scattiness

thyme

Thymus vulgaris

AVOID DURING PREGNANCY

Method of extraction	Steam distillation of the leaves and flowers
Enhances	Self-confidence, calmness, balance, focus, concentration, happiness, satisfaction, vitality, healing, determination
Reduces	Depression, fatigue, nervous exhaustion, colds and flu, fear, insomnia, anxiety, insect repellent

valerian

Valeriana officinalis

Method of extraction	Steam distillation of the root
Enhances	Calmness, happiness, emotional release, moving on, relaxation, deep sleep

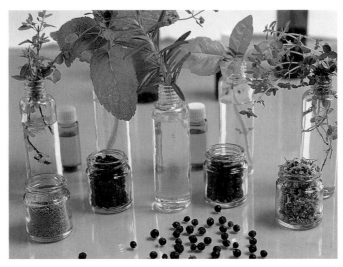

Reduces	Stress, depression, anger, aggression, hysteria, insomnia, addiction

vanilla
Vanilla plantifolia

Enhances	Positive energy, uplifting, sensuality, romance
Reduces	Insecurity, boredom, sexual apathy

vetiver
Vetiveria zizanioides

Method of extraction	Steam distillation of the dried roots
Enhances	Wisdom, emotional release, self-confidence, centring, security, sensuality, love, comfort, emotional strength, inner wisdom, intuition, serenity
Reduces	Stress, nervous exhaustion, premenstrual stress, sleeping difficulties, over-sensitivity, vulnerability, fear, emotional burdens, scattiness, anxiety, loss of direction, stagnation, self-doubt, anger

ylang ylang
Cananga odorata

Method of extraction	Steam distillation of the flower petals
Enhances	Sensuality, exuberance, warmth, self-confidence, openness, joy, acceptance, relaxation, serenity, togetherness, tenderness
Reduces	Depression, sleeping difficulties, nervous tension, premenstrual stress, sexual inadequacy, frustration, moodiness, guilt, rigidity, thoughtlessness, broken heart

index

credits

The author would like to thank all the companies who donated their products for use in the photography for this book.

page vi, top
Teapot and tea bowls from Made in Japan; oil burner from The Body Shop

page vii, middle and bottom
Oil burners from Jurlique, The Body Shop and Sanctum

page x, top
Oil burner from Sanctum

page xi, top and middle
Bottles and containers from The Bottle People

bottom
Celestial body and bath oil and soap from Venustus; Aquatherapy bath salts from Aveda; soap dish from Authentics; shaving brush from Jurlique; oil burner from Sanctum

pages 1 and 6
Teapot and tea bowls from Made in Japan; oil burner from The Body Shop

page 5
Bottle from The Bottle People

pages 9 and 11
Bottle from The Bottle People; soap dish from Authentics; soap from The Body Shop

pages 12 and 16
Oil burner from Sanctum

page 47
Bottles from The Bottle People

page 53
Oil burner from The Body Shop
Bottles from The Bottle People

page 68
Container from The Bottle People

page 70
Oil burners from Jurlique and Sanctum

page 74
Bottles from The Bottle People

page 89
Clarity night serum, Sacred shower gel, Tahitian body and bath oil, Serenity floral water from Venustus; soaps and bath ball from Lush; oil burner from Jurlique

page 91
Clarity night serum, Sacred shower gel, Tahitian body and bath oil, Serenity floral water from Venustus; soaps and bath ball from Lush

page 96
Oil burners from Jurlique, Sanctum and The Body Shop

page 103
Oil burner from Venustus

page 106
Clarity night serum, Sacred shower gel, Tahitian body and bath oil, Serenity floral water from Venustus; soaps and bath ball from Lush

pages 111 and 114
Oil burner from Jurlique

page 118
Container from The Bottle People

page 123
Celestial body and bath oil and soap from Venustus; Aquatherapy bath salts from Aveda; soap dish and pump bottle from Authentics; shaving kit from Jurlique, oil burner from Sanctum

page 127
Celestial body and bath oil from Venustus; pump bottle from Authentics; razor from Jurlique

page 133
Container from The Bottle People; oil burner from Sanctum; Aveda bath bar

page 134
Container from The Bottle People; Aveda bath bar

pages 141 and 142
Bottles from The Bottle People

page 149
Platter from Rice; chopsticks and green bowl from Made in Japan

page 156
Bowl from Made in Japan

page 182
Bottles from The Bottle People

List of suppliers of pure essential oils in Australia

AVEDA
58–60 Easey Street, Collingwood,
Melbourne, Victoria 3066
(03) 9419 3355

ESSENTIAL THERAPEUTICS
Head Office, 56–60 Easey Street,
Collingwood, Melbourne,
Victoria 3066
(03) 9419 7711

IN ESSENCE
Head Office, 221 Kerr Street,
Fitzroy, Melbourne, Victoria 3065
(03) 9899 9266

JURLIQUE INTERNATIONAL
Head Office, PO Box 522,
Mount Barker, South Australia 5251
(08) 8391 0577

RED EARTH
Head Office, 66 Leicester Street,
Carlton, Melbourne, Victoria 3053
(03) 9347 2666

SANCTUM PURE BODY PRODUCTS
75 Epping Road, North Ryde,
New South Wales 2113
(02) 9888 6333

SPRINGFIELDS
Unit 2/2 Anella Avenue, Castle
Hill, New South Wales 2154
(02) 9894 9933

SUNSPIRIT OILS
PO Box 85, Byron Bay,
New South Wales 2481
(02) 6685 6333

THE BODY SHOP
Head Office, cnr Wellington and
Jacksons Roads, Mulgrave,
Melbourne, Victoria 3170
(03) 9565 0500

VENUSTUS
381 Oxford Street, Paddington,
New South Wales 2021
(02) 9361 4014

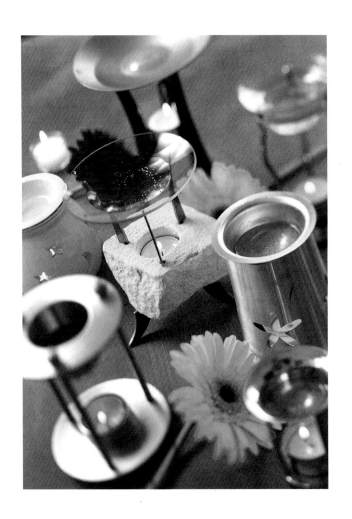